THE
FORGOTTEN
FOUR
FLAVOURS
DIET

ELIAS KEFALIDIS

CONTENTS

INTRODUCTION

Do you know why you are fat? Do you know why you can't lose weight? Do you know who is to blame for you being in a deadlock and continuously occupied with diets and health foods? The person who is to blame is in your house, and you can't do anything to her – it's your mother. Because of her ignorance or because of following the fashion of the time, she has accustomed you to eating 'flavours' that are 'killing' you. These are found in foods that act like drugs, and with each passing day, they are shortening instead of lengthening your life.

You will no doubt question whether it is possible that a mother would wish to harm her child. In fact, she does – in the same you harm your child. Nutrition is the most fundamental lesson that should, ideally, be taught before the onset of pregnancy, or at least as soon as pregnancy is confirmed – because from the moment of pregnancy, the embryo is exposed to flavours. According to research, our predilection for various flavours derives from our mothers, and if a mother's diet is based on sweet or salty processed foodstuffs, it creates problems in embryonic development which later lead to obesity and other illnesses. Later, when the child starts on liquid and later still on solid foods, it learns and becomes accustomed to certain flavours to the extent that it develops a dependency on them. And which flavours are these? Again, it's the sweet and salty flavours. What mother ever experimented in the first or second year – as should be done – to introduce her child to sweet and salty flavours? And by this, I don't mean squashing a whole lemon in the baby's cream or feeding it on ground greens with their roots still attached. In this way, the phenomenon of nutritional neophobia appears, that is – a fear to try new flavours. Consequently, the child is fed on potatoes, spaghetti, bread like foodstuffs, and snacks.

In adolescence, the child's nutrition is undertaken by the food industry which reinforces incorrect nutritional choices. As a result of ready meals and teenager snacks, the child's weight increases and makes the child a lifelong prisoner of sweet and salty flavours: the solution to this problem is – the dietician.

And what exactly is a dietician? The majority of those dieticians that I have met are people who chose to become dieticians rather than teachers, army officers, musicians, or actors. It is, namely, a profession which provides certain recipes by which fat patients can lose weight.

My experience at the hands of dieticians – which I describe in chapter 1 – is truly tragic. During the course of 30 years of dieting, I expected to get a recipe – exactly what they advertised, incidentally – that would help me to lose weight. Nobody taught me that the prescription for slimming is healthy eating: to be careful of what I eat and what is best for my health. Everybody used to follow the successful diet formulas of the times. I must say that some of the many diets that I followed had as their goal my rapid loss of weight – but this doesn't happen in nature. The brain doesn't allow the loss of weight without reason or just because you suddenly want to look nice. On the contrary, if the body experiences health problems, it functions differently.

So, the specialists took control of me – giving me specific 'prescriptions' and trying to get me to lose weight. They had divided the slimming process into two phases: the first phase was concerned with losing weight, and the second phase was concerned with sustenance. Now, that's something I have never un-derstood. Why did I have to partake in the first stage? Was it just to exhaust my body both mentally and physically, after which the only thing that I wanted was to regain the weight that I had lost?

In my case, I have been dieting for thirty years. If every YEAR I lost only two kilos, I should have lost sixty kilos by now. And from the 127 kilos I got to as a result of the diets, I should weigh sixty-seven kilos – a miracle! But diets fail – and for many reasons: they neglect taste and the dynamic effect that it has on foods; they are programmes which must produce rapid results; they concentrate on how much people eat rather than why they eat; they set unrealistic goals; they maintain old habits; they create myths about miraculous foods; they search for the ideal results on the basis of the ideal number of kilos; and they fail because nobody has ever explained to you in depth that you will have to diet for the WHOLE of your life.

The problem that I talk about in chapter 2 is how sweet and salty flavours have become 'national dishes' in a lot of countries. Thus, without knowing, we accustom ourselves to these flavours and as a result we are led closer and closer to obesity and the loss of health.

A series of researches report addiction caused by sugar is greater than that caused by hard drugs: even drugs such as heroin and cocaine. Indeed, some scientists believe that supplementary sugar intake reaches levels that are at the limits of toxicity.

Sauces, soups, chocolates, biscuits, sweets, bread, desserts, soft drinks, ice-cream, snacks, flour, spaghetti and pasta products, sausages and cold cooked meats, dairy products, processed frozen foods, marmalades and jams, and many other related foodstuffs have a prominent presence in supermarkets. The sweet flavour – that is sugar – goes under many different names that we are not aware of when shopping sugar containing foodstuffs. It often appears on the labels of packaged foods as one of the following names: lactose, glucose, dextrose, malt extract, castor sugar, invert sugar, isoglucose, brown sugar, lactose, maltose, maltodextrin, molasses, agave nectar, sucrose, glucose syrup, syrup or cane juice, brown sugar syrup, rice syrup, fructose corn syrup, modified starch, and fructose.

And if what is on the supermarket shelves is not sweet, then it is salty. These choices contribute and cause illnesses in addition to obesity, for example: hypertension, diabetes, heart problems, and cancer – exactly those illnesses that people die from nowadays. And all these foods are based on the notion of delicious flavor. So, how do foodstuffs become appetizing?

They become appetizing when the flavour is intensified and when additives are included: such additives can be found in all foodstuffs. Snacking is 'criminalized', but it is those chemicals that also produce a pleasant sensation in alcoholic drinks, chewing gum, sweets that enhance the appearance of mushrooms, roots, bulbs and tubers, and nuts. They are also used for spicing red meats, poultry, game, and fish.

Acids are also used for many purposes in the food industry. They are used for improving the raw materials used in the confectionery industry, and in foodstuffs such as canned fruit and vegetables, fruit juices, marmalades and jams, pasta foods, and chocolates. They are used for improving food colouring in foodstuffs such as jellies, mustards, instant soups, soft drinks, margarine, oil, butter, and cheese. They are also used as additives for making foodstuffs softer or crunchier. Finally, additive enzymes and seasonings are used in bread, diet products, and buns. The catalogue of uses is enormous.

Indeed, the problem is so serious that in 2003 the WHO (World Health Organization) issued a recommendation that the daily intake of sugar should equal not more than 10% of the daily number of calories. And what was the result? In many countries, the average daily consumption of sugar actually reached 25% of the daily number of calories. So in 2014, the WHO returned with a new limit: setting a limit of 5% on the daily consumption of sugar. This was probably after the enormous amount of research on the evils of sweet flavours. But that's crazy! The 10% level didn't produce any results, so why should the 5% level?

However, there is a solution, and that is discussed in the chapter 3. Three areas in Greece have the same basis for their diets: Crete, Ikaria, and Mount Athos. This diet includes the four flavours and is a holistic system that originated in ancient Greece: it is a diet that on the one hand attempts to regenerate the body and on the other hand seeks to limit illnesses. Characteristically flavoured foods that were eaten in the Minoan era in Crete, in ancient Sparta, and in ancient Athens have been forgotten. Nowadays, such foods would be classified as superfoods. In the Greece of today, the four flavors diet is only followed by the inhabitants of rural areas who are reluctant to abandon their traditional diet.

Some of these rural communities have been medically monitored and have presented unique findings concerning the health and longevity of the inhabitants. One area of particular interest is the Greek island of Crete.

Since 1960, specialists have reported on the diet of the inhabitants of the Greek island of Crete: it is from here that the so-called Mediterranean diet evolved. Since 2009, people have been talking about the miracle of Ikaria where the inhabitants – just don't seem to die. You may also like to know that the diet of the monks of Mount Athos has remained unchanged for 1,000 years – no, you haven't misread it: one thousand years!

The inhabitants of these three areas have – with the exception of some minor regional variations – the same diet. Furthermore, they don't feed themselves on processed foods, and they neither fill the table with junk food nor do they exclude different flavours.

Their diet includes the following foodstuffs:

Cultivated and natural (bitter) salads,
Legumes (sweet)
Fruit (bitter, sour, sweet)
Wild greens (bitter)
Fish (sweet)
Raw olive oil (bitter)
Olives (bitter)
Meat (sweet)
Dairy products (sour, salty, sweet)
Wine (bitter, sweet)
Greek coffee (bitter)
Beverages (bitter) and
Herbs (bitter)

Furthermore, due to religious traditions, in the three regions previously mentioned, fasting occurs on every other day: they consume Greek foodstuffs on 195 days of the year and on the remaining 170 days eat bread, greens, boiled vegetables, fruits, legumes, nuts, and tahini. A perfect detoxification experience for the human body.

Additionally, in all three of these regions, herbs are used on a daily basis in the preparation of meals, salads, and beverages. These have high nutritional value, and they contribute through detoxification and other functions in confronting many disorders, as well as fine tuning the body. Indeed, as research and the many decades of experience in Greece have shown: the regular use of beverages (dittany, siderite, marjoram, mint, pennyroyal, etc.) can give modern humans optimal health and well-being.

Additionally, they are rich in active substances, and a lot of them react positively against cancer, obesity, hypertension, Alzheimer's disease, heart problems, and diabetes. They also strengthen the immune system, help in detoxification, and they have a positive effect on the kidneys. By the way – all these herbs have a taste ranging from mild to very bitter. Is this just fortuitous?

I'm surprised that after 30 years of dieting – no specialist had ever included herbs in my slimming program; after all, herbs have zero calories and are rich in antioxidants. Instead, the specialists let me drink coffees, and in moderation: juices, and alcoholic beverages.

It is characteristic that when some region of Greece changes diet and switches to two flavours – something that happens amongst the younger generations – the inhabitants of that region start to get fat and manifest the ailments associated with western diets. That is why – according to an OECD report – Greek boys and girls in the 5 – 17 age group are 'champions' in obesity in. Moreover, according to a recent OECD (Organization for Economic Cooperation and Development) report, the life expectancy of the Greeks, which in the 1970s was one of the highest in Europe, has since fallen to the 20th position among the thirty-four member countries of the OECD.

In chapter 4, I describe how I discovered the problem with my diet (which was the consumption of only sweet and salty tasting foods), and how I put into practice the four flavours diet. Being honest with yourself, have you realized the power that flavours have on your diet? Do you think that you would eat more if you didn't have the sense of taste? When you are ill and have lost your taste, do you eat with pleasure? Or perhaps do you just eat mechanically while waiting for your sense of taste to return so that you can once again enjoy lots of food?

That, then, is the great secret. Taste is the vehicle for consuming quantities of sweet and salty foods.

And when I refer to the four flavours diet, I am referring in particular to those taste buds that are stimulated by raw food because when they are cooked with different sauces, spices and herbs they taste different to the foods in the raw state, for example: fruit can be sour, or sweet, but not very bitter; greens are mainly bitter as are herbs; meat and fish are sweet as are legumes.

As for bread, you have to assign it to the relevant category: a sweet bread, bread with salt (salty), and sourdough bread (sour). The same applies to cheese: it can be sweet, salty, or sour. Historically, there are four principal food flavours: bitter, sweet, sour, and salty. Hot and spicy/pungent tasting foods do not represent a particular flavour but rather, the body's response to certain chemical compounds. The same applies to astringent flavoured foods, because we realize their effects after ingestion.

The four flavours diet allows you to eat every kind of foodstuff, but in moderation. For example: fruit, vegetables, meat, fish, legumes, dairy products, cereals, and herbs. By the criteria of the four flavours diet, you wouldn't only eat sweet tasting fruit, but sour fruit as well. You wouldn't eat a salad with only meat, but also with cereals, or with cheese, or with legumes, or with fish. On this diet, you don't eat much protein or too much starch. You don't nourish yourself on just a few foods – but with all the variety that natural foods offer.

THE FIRST THING I did (disheartened by diets) was to keep a log of flavours, that is – a record of what I ate every day. In my log I recorded the flavors and my eating habits: this showed me that the dominant flavors were, on the whole, sweet and salty.
Here are some of the foods which I consume on a daily basis: white bread, sandwiches, brioche, sliced bread, burgers, meats with various sauces (sweet and bitter-sweet), cheese, pasta foods with various sauces, pizzas, milkshakes, cakes, crisps, shrimps, croissants, chocolates, and ice creams. When you understand what you eat and your brain registers it, then you will eat properly – and only when you're hungry.

THE SECOND thing that I did was to substitute processed sweets with natural sweets, and salt with salt and herbs. In this way, I stopped eating cereals, biscuits, doughnuts, buns, cakes, croissants, and pancakes with jam – and replaced them all with Greek yoghurt topped with honey, or with a few raisins, or 4-5 dried fruits, or with fresh sweet fruits such as bananas, pears, and apples. I must admit – I didn't miss the sweet foods at all. Moreover, desserts are not a necessary foodstuff for survival: they form a modern eating habit which loads us with calories. As it concerns my consumption of salt, I substituted a mixture of salt and herbs (80% Mediterranean herbs and 20% unrefined salt) for plain salt. Later on, I also replaced that with a variety of herbs. In all honesty – I didn't miss salt at all. After all, we can obtain it from cheese, bread, and many other foods too. I also substituted water and Greek herbal beverages (a lot of herbs, though) for soft drinks.

THE THIRD thing I did was correct my breakfast and dinner: instead of just eating foods with sweet and salty flavours, I tried foods with the other two flavours. I can recommend some recipes for breakfast and dinner that have all four flavours.

THE FOURTH thing I did was to change my lunch by enriching it with bitter and sour flavours. Eating foods with the four flavours made me feel complete, nutritionally speaking.

Finally, I stress the size of the plate (which contained food with the four flavors) that I ate on in the morning, at midday, or in the evening: this is important because the size of the plate is a measure of the amount of food. In this way, I was able to control the amount that I ate.

In the book there are recipes and a table with foods listed under the headings: sweet, bitter, salty, and sour. You can add your own flavours to these, and make your own diet programme for breakfast, and lunch or dinner.

It's a fact that I started without anxiety to lose kilos and not to put on kilos – and do you know why? It's because I am losing kilos as if I were in the weight maintenance phase. I don't rush myself; I don't inflict stress on my body, and I eat foods with all flavours: by doing these things, I have found my equilibrium.

On top of that – and after the ups and downs in the price of triglycerides – my diabetes, cholesterol, pain in the knees, and middle back pain have all started little by little to improve because of the four flavours diet.

As it concerns exercising, you don't need to while away all day in the gym as if you were training for special forces. I exercise thirty minutes a day by quick walking. We need to build up our hands and legs. If you think about it, we only need to spend half an hour out of twenty-four hours on exercising. The other twenty-three and a half hours will be spent moving from your bed to your office chair then to your sofa and back to bed again.

CHAPTER 1
THE EXPERIENCE

"PREJUDICE" LEAD ME TO DIETING

It's winter, and it it's raining, and I'm getting ready for a business appointment. Oh! How I hate my clothes. I'd like them to be wide, but they mustn't. This suit I am trying on is comfortable, but the white shirt is tight. So now I am looking in the wardrobe, and although there's another white shirt of a different style – that's far too wide! I've reached an impasse! Once again, I don't know what to wear. I curse to myself because I just can't get slim. I look out of the window – it's pouring down! I'll have to take an umbrella too, and by the time I get into the car I'll be drenched because I didn't park the car near the house last night: I wanted to walk – so I parked it far away.

At last, I opt for the tight shirt. It's awful, but nothing else can be done because for my size of stomach there are no appropriately sized clothes. So here I am with my stomach extruding outwards and my jacket 'floating' on my body. I pick up my bag and leave.

Having got into the car, I discover that I can't move. I feel as if I have been placed in a press: I feel as if I am being squeezed by some external force. Sitting in the car, I feel that my trousers are comfortable, but my stomach – it's suffocating me. I can't breathe. Suddenly, I am seized with terror at the thought of what I will look like to the company president. I am a nineteen year old trainee journalist and I am on the go from 8 am to 11 pm. I try not to think about my clothes because I'll have to see the day through dressed like this. I start to perspire – even though I know it's only 15ºC.

Fortunately, I arrive on time at the company. I get out of the car and tuck in my shirt which has already started to creep out of my trousers. I pull in my stomach in order to appear more 'normal', but I seriously wonder about how long I can hold it in. I feel as if I am deep sea diving although I don't know what it's really like for someone who weighs 127 kilos, but divers must probably feel something like this when their oxygen is running out.

Whatever! I'm now standing outside the lift trying to collect my thoughts, and people are starting to crowd around me: but because of my anxiety about my shirt, and the tight tie – once again, I didn't manage to tie the knot without strangling myself – I can't turn.

At last the lift arrives, and we all get in. In the lift I catch a glimpse of another two forty-five to fifty year old women; a tall, slim twenty-five to thirty year old man cuddled up in the corner; a bald man of about forty; and another man who is about fifty. The appointment is on the sixth floor, and we are now on the third floor when the lift suddenly – stops. It just hangs there motionless. They all start to look at each other – but no one says anything. At some point, I look up, and I get the sensation that everyone is looking at me as if to say, "Hey, fatso! You count for three people. Why did you come in with us?" I start to sweat. I feel as if I'm in a Turkish bath. I wipe away the sweat which is pouring out of me. The lift telephone was working initially, so it was possible to inform the technical people of our situation before it stopped working – but I felt suffocated. I felt as if everyone was against me. With the exception of the tall man, all of us were overweight: they all had their 'flab', but they were all looking disdainfully at me. These few minutes of 'imprisonment' really seemed endless.

The president had learnt about the details of what had happened and was waiting for me with some orange juice, water, and pastries. I entered the room in a flushed state. He saw that I had reached my tether. Although he invited me to remove my jacket, I didn't dare to take it off as I could feel my shirt completely stuck to my body.

I don't even recall what he was asking me. I tried to finish as quickly as possible because my mind was still preoccupied with the aggressive way in which the people in the lift had been looking at me. What can I say – you get 'prejudice' even in a lift.

As if it isn't enough that everywhere they 'persecute' you, or look at you derisively if you have a few extra kilos – soon they won't even allow us into lifts.

I got into the car and headed off to work, but all I could think of was dieting: whether quick results diets or slow results diets – it was only diets that I was thinking about.

I arrived at work and handed in my article, but my thoughts were stuck on 'prejudice' – what an irony! The world of mass media – the influential and the fashion setters – recommends a world of slim people. But each year people are getting fatter, and those same people in the mass media publish statistics on the increase in obesity. Why, then, is it ugly only when we see somebody who is overweight, but it is not the same or even worse when we see someone who is thin and bald? The figure of a bald person is incredibly funny. I mean, don't all bald people look cartoon-like? Their heads shine like toilet titles: but this is acceptable. Why should the physical appearance of a tall, slim person be acceptable? Have you noticed how tall people walk? They drag their feet and they bend in the middle. Doesn't the sight of someone who can't accommodate their body make you laugh? Yet, such people are accepted. I have the impression that fatness, baldness, thinness, and tallness are not contagious diseases. But form the foregoing – it's only fatness that is persecuted. And, please, don't talk to me about matters concerned with health. The 'prejudice' directed against fat people isn't because others wish fat people to be healthy. They don't look at my microbiological tests when they charge me for my excess weight when I travel by plane. It follows that I shouldn't travel as much as I smoke: years which would usually be associated with a severe medical history.

I want to unwind. I want to up root from within me the beast of obesity that has settled itself in my mind and shows no signs of wanting to leave. I feel like a third, or fourth, or even fifth class citizen.

I reach my den – my room – since I live with my parents. The first thing I think about is getting a good meal and drinking a glass of wine. Shall I take revenge, namely, against myself? Maybe. The next day, I am thinking about going on a strict diet: since the age of nineteen, I have undergone dozens of diets in the last thirty years: some with a dietician, some without, named and unnamed, alone, and as a member of a group. The results have been disheartening: I lost weight then I put on weigh; then I lost weight and then put on weight again – and so forth. My daily routine was an ordeal, and my psychological well-being had hit rock bottom. Let's have a look at my tragic experience and some of the numerous diets that I had undergone all those years and which produced no results for me, but for others – maybe.

1 WEIGHT WATCHER – *The 'apotheosis' of the portion*
I remember – when I was nineteen – a red balance that was calibrated in grams, and how my mother used to try to prepare the little helpings. I didn't feel as if I was eating, but rather – just snacking. I couldn't wait to eat because it was the pleasure of the little helping, and it was something completely foreign for a fat boy like me: but – I gave it up.

2 NASA DIETS – *You melt quickly! You stop quickly!*
The sooner I felt that I was losing weight the quicker I had a mental block, and I wanted to stop as soon as the scales stuck. Every day I had two eggs for breakfast – and sometimes at lunch I had two eggs again. I became obsessed with this matter. Because of work, I read that too many eggs are bad for you: later I read in some researches that the harmful effects were imputed to the yolk only, and in other researches that there was no harm at all, and so forth. For example, boxers, wrestlers, and weightlifters must be of a certain weight for their category; otherwise, they will have to compete in different weight category.

I started on this diet and the result was really rapid: I felt myself changing quickly. On the one hand it filled me with joy; on the other hand, though, it was something strange for me. I didn't know this programme at all. After many days, I ceased to lose weight, and I also quickly became disappointed. My feelings were spontaneous, and I couldn't get used to them; I couldn't make the change mine. Where I needed strengthening, I found myself alone with the eggs and the meats. I started to crack. Since I was eating the same foods but wasn't losing weight, I started to add other foods, and then after that – I quit.

3 LOVE DIET – *I got slim because I was happy*

This is the first diet that I didn't feel that I was actually dieting because my mind was elsewhere. I was getting on well with my girlfriend, and I decided to feel even better by losing some weight. So I asked a dietician to put me on a diet based on traditional Greek foods. Indeed, he gave me the programme; I paid him, and we arranged for an appointment in two weeks' time. The menu consisted of fresh beans or legumes or stuffed vegetables and a piece of feta cheese: alternatively, the same diet but with a piece of moussaka or a piece of pasticcio. This was to be eaten without bread or a salad, and meat or fish with salad were to be eaten twice a week only.

I must say, it was the first time that dieting had appeared to be so easy: the meals were the best I could eat; the quantities, I can say, even reached the size of large portions. I was sure that I was going to succeed; I was full of unbelievable self-confidence.

Because I felt nice, the last thing that I had on my mind was food – and that's why I lost fifteen kilos in five months. And what's more, the success of this effort was received enthusiastically by my girlfriend. She showed me that she could empathize with me and that she wanted me to continue. And I did – until we broke up.

4 ATKINS DIET – *The meat eater's delight*

I had put on weight again, and I had this arsehole reporter for a boss who kept on reminding me of it. Almost every day was a war of nerves, so I started on the Atkins diet, which was fashionable at the time. It actually reminded me a lot of the NASA diet. Because I was eating a lot of meat again, it was a relatively easy diet to follow and it produced rapid results – but it made me feel like a butcher's son.

Moreover, the diet was additional to what I normally ate, and it was a mechanical and monotonous programme; in other words, I was bored when I was eating. Food is supposed to be all about flavour, pleasure, and imagination. If I change beef for chicken and chicken for pork, something's not all right. I ate because I had to eat and in that way I would lose weight. Again, I felt that if I were to stop,

I would put on weight – something that actually happened as soon as I started to eat all the foodstuffs.

5 ALTERNATIVE DIET – *A therapist, a guru, a Zulu*

In my attempt to lose weight, I resorted to a dietician of great fame who was well-known in both the traditional and alternative dieting circles in Athens. Resolute in the belief that I was embarking on something different, I entered the ground floor of a pleasant two-storey house. Like any fat person, I was I was looking for a reason to hang on. When I got in, a young lady took my details and requested me to take my shoes off and leave them outside in the hall. I obeyed. On entering a small lounge, I was met by a sea of multi-colored socks, and flabby people. After a while the dietician came in and started to measure me with a tailor's tape measure – I kid you not! He measured the width of my back, and the distance from my shoulder diagonally across to my stomach while dictating instructions to his assistant who was busy writing them down. He then weighed me on a small weigh-bridge like those one finds in transport depots. The whole procedure was accompanied by a series of ah's as the dietician expressed his surprise at some fact or other. The only actual words that I actually heard him utter were, "Strong constitution" – and that was when he struck me on the sternum. His breath stank as if he hadn't eaten for days; fortunately, he didn't talk a lot. Anyway, the diet sheet that he gave me was for a seven day period. I had to eat the following foods for the first four days:

MORNING: 2 bananas

LUNCH: 300 g boiled potatoes with 2 – 3 soupspoons of oil, lemon, salt, and oregano

EVENING + NIGHT: 2 fruit juices each of 150 ml

There were also two instructions:

CHEWING: chew each mouthful 20 times

FLUIDS: restrict your intake to the bare minimum. Half a litre a day

On the fifth day: two fruit juices and water, but on the other two days – which fell on the weekend – only water. Having booked the next appointment, I left without hope. Inside me, I was sure that I would never come back again, and indeed – I didn't. For the record, I managed to comply with the first four days: I ate the potatoes in the morning; I took the bananas with me to eat later, and at night I drank the fruit juices. In the end the result was hardship, hunger, and disappointment.

6 BLOOD GROUP DIETS – *I was on another blood group's diet*

I had a really good laugh with this diet, and I still laugh my head off when I think about it. This was because the diet that was appropriate for my blood group was inconsistent with what I was eating at home. In other words, I was a different man in another person's body while belonging to blood group O which characterized me as a hunter – a carnivore who should have been eating meat and exercising. But a typical Greek home cooks meat only once every fifteen days: the other days it consumes fish, legumes, and cooked food with vegetables prepared in a saucepan – which after medical research became known as the "Mediterranean Diet". So, although I was blood group O, I had become accustomed to eating the food of blood group A. How could I possibly consume large amounts of meat as I was not use to it? Something was not right. Oh, well! I quit again.

7 A GENUINELY WISE DIET – *Forget the dietician and listen to the Cretan's wise words*

A genuinely wise diet. The apotheosis of a wise lifestyle – not the diet. I started off on an express diet, but I ended up being influenced by the advice of a wise Cretan. A group of about thirty of us decided to spend a fortnight at a guest house near Mount Ida in Crete.

With my mind absorbed with Crete, I started on a diet which promised that I would lose nine kilos in two weeks – but I only lost three and a half kilos. The rationale behind this diet is based on deprivation, namely: in the morning herbal beverages and maybe half a glass of juice; at midday the celebrated 120 grams of meat or fish with vegetables; and in the evening the same. You have to drink a lot of water, and walk a lot – if you can endure it and are still standing at the end of the day. In spite of all that, this was the second time that a diet hadn't disturbed me, and that was because of two things:

1. I knew it wasn't a life-long programme – just a fortnight.

2. I felt refreshed and satisfied with the material goods I had acquired at my age – confirmation, you see – and the trip was uppermost in my mind.

I lost weight, got ready and then I left. We reached the island and we drove it to where we were going to stay. I was really impressed by the people I saw: people over sixty-five years old walking briskly, or climbing hills, or working in fields with the flexibility a child. I had read many things about the Cretan diet, and the researches on regional longevity. But now I had seen something truly sensational with my own eyes. I was genuinely impressed. As soon as we arrived, we split up into three or four groups. Some wanted to wake up early, some late, and others wanted to go for a swim at noon. Some wanted to eat only once a day and drink beverages, others wanted to eat twice a day. I avoided getting involved in this chaos because I wanted to go swimming in the morning – when there would be few people about to see by big belly. When the others woke up, I would go out and visit a few cafes in order to get to know the place.

And that's how things went. After two days, we got into a routine: during the day, everyone did whatever they wanted to, and in the evenings we would all get together. In the mornings, I would drink Greek coffee at the guest house while marveling at Mount Ida. It was there I made the acquaintance of the owner's father: the sixty-eight year old captain Manouso, who just couldn't sit still for a moment; he always had to be doing something. When at times I used to call him to drink a few glasses of raki, he would reply in the local dialect, "Are you mad? Get up and do some work."

"If you don't move yourself, you won't see a good day," he used to say to me. Wise captain Manouso had a philosophical explanation for everything: for what he is going to eat; for how long he is going to sleep; and for which things he can do in the course of a day. He was active, but he didn't have anxiety. And when he was having a plate of food and a little salad, it was as if he were having the most expensive dish.

He ate slowly and with concentration; he didn't chit-chat with the others nearby him. In fact, when we first met, his wife had made three Cretan dishes and invited me to come and eat with them. Captain Manousos choose which food he was going to you eat with his salad. I tucked into everything – I just couldn't stop myself. But captain Manousos caused me to stop when he said to me, "Food isn't meant for filling up our bellies; it's meant for maintaining our bodies." No sooner had he said this than my spoon froze. I immediately lost my appetite.

Over the course of the next few days, I decided to follow captain Manousos in everything that he did: to copy his daily routine. It was entertaining because this indefatigable man sensed my confirmation and enthusiasm, and he treated me like a son. Little by little, I too began to feel lighter and more ethereal. In the beginning, I thought that it was competitiveness that had swept me off my feet. Later on, I realized what had happened when my friends saw me and said, "I thought you dieted before we came here, so you could eat here. And now you are still continuing on your diet?" But I hadn't understood it. In my ears I could hear the deep voice of captain Manousos: "Food isn't for filling up, but for maintenance."

The holiday had come to an end; before leaving, we bid farewell to the people we had got to know, and I bid captain Manousos goodbye. My greatest anxiety was to find out how much I weighed. I stood staring with bulging eyes at the scales: I had lost three kilos in fifteen days. The strange thing is that I don't know how it happened.

8 VEGETARIAN DIETS – *They aren't diets; it's detoxification*
This was a diet that turned out not to be a diet – but detoxification. I had become an editor of a medical journal, and among the columns of print there was a proposal for an alternative therapy. On the day that I was first introduced to

my colleagues, the author of article was also present. I discussed several work related issues with him, and later we talked about the medical aspects of obesity. We talked for quite a while: I explained my problem to him, and he suggested that I see an alternative doctor (for the second time, by the way). This doctor gave me a diet that included lots of fresh fruit, and vegetable juices, and a lot of salads. He also forbade meat, dairy products, cheese, and bread. I left stunned. Throughout the whole journey home, all I could think about was – what's left to eat: salads and fruit? I started with great difficulty, but the truth is that I did not feel it weighing on me.

The day came when the doctor, my colleague at work, submitted his article for the medical journal. After work, I requested him to advise me about my diet: "If I put it into practice, will it adversely affect my health? How can I possibly feel better if I will only be eating a minimum of foodstuffs?"

He just asked me one thing, "Why do you want to go on this diet?"

"To lose weight, of course," I replied. To which he responded: "Look, if you only eat those foods, you are sure to lose weight. But it would be better, though, not to start with that diet. This vegetarian diet is mainly for detoxification, but you will still definitely lose weight. Nevertheless, I don't recommend it; you will also have to take nutritional supplements daily because this is not a complete diet." So, before I had even properly started – I quit.

9 SAFE FOOD DIETS – *The joy of life style*

After numerous diets and a lot of reading, I decided to try a medical institute that specialized in actually monitoring obesity by the use of the most modern equipment in the field of medicine.

The environment at the institute was something between an advertising agency and a multinational corporation. All the members of the staff were beautiful and slim: the only people who were fat – were the patients. And they were the only people that went there. They interviewed me; they informed me of the costs (around €700 in total), and that I would have to submit to a series of medical examinations. These examinations would not only include the standard medical tests such as cholesterol level, and triglyceride blood tests, but also other tests such as tests to measure the quantity of body fat, and apnea.

I did the tests, and I was informed by the competent member of staff about the condition of my body: my metabolism was blocked. He then explained the system that would be used to resolve this problem – it was their discovery.
It included breakfast, brunch, lunch, tea, and dinner. The foodstuffs that constituted the diet were those with the highest nutritional values, namely: the more nutritious and less harmful meats; and the most nutritious and non starchy vegetables. The same criteria were applied to fruits and nuts.

As soon as I saw what they were giving me to eat – I complained. I said to the doctor, "I think it's a lot. I don't eat so much." He replied, "What are you talking about…? We are going to unblock your body, and the problem of obesity will be removed. But you will have to faithfully apply the diet."

I started eating exactly what they told me to, and I noticed that I was beginning to bloat. When the day of the interview arrived – after a fortnight – I discovered that I had put on one kilo and 100 grams.

With a stern expression on his face, he said to me, "We stressed that you should not do whatever comes into your mind, but faithfully implement the program." I couldn't take any more. Raising my voice too, (having been so frustrated by the experience of so many diets) I replied, "Well, since I'm eating more now than before, it's logical, isn't it?"

If I hadn't been able to control my temper, we would have ended up fighting there and then. He gave me the programme for the following fortnight and left in a right state. I then simply thought about doing the diet at my own pace, namely: three and not five meals a day.

The day of the next rendezvous arrived. He weighs me and finds that I have lost two kilos. Then with a sweet expression on his face, he says, "Can you now see what the result is when you faithfully follow the programme?" I controlled myself from… I took the next programme and – I quit, again. I had lost a month's effort, and my mental health.

10 EXTRA HELPINGS DIET – *A little food but lots of extra helpings*

Disappointed with everything and as my weight had reached 127 kilos, for the first time – I actually wanted to go on a diet. All this time, I had been eating just for the sake of satiety, and I was sick of all those experts, and all those well-known and lesser known diets. Well, one day, a friend of mine at work left a note on my desk with the telephone number of a holistic doctor. As soon as I saw it, I became furious. "Another waste of time, again!" I thought to myself. But the problem was that I couldn't sleep at night: I had to struggle, and I was lucky if I could manage to get four or five hours of continuous sleep.

It was this insomnia that eventually forced me to go – so I booked an appointment. The doctor's surgery was decorated in an Indian style (Asian Indian). So, the doctor calls me into his office, and the first thing he gets me to do is to hold a piece of metal, I think it was a piece of copper, in one hand while he tapped on the tips of my fingernails with a pointed instrument. According to the level of my 'toxicity' – well, that's what he said – the instrument would record a score ranging from 0 (pure) to 10 (highly toxic): all my reading were very close to ten.

He then used one of those instruments that eye-specialists use to check the irises. "Just for conformation," he said. Ah! On completion of my examination and looking at me with a stern expression, he informed me that – I was in a very bad condition. My body had aged and I needed detoxification. He explained that first of all the bowels had to be cleaned and then he would start to build up my health. He wrote down what I had to eat, but for faster results – according to him – I would also have to take various supplements for two months: after which, he would review the situation.

Conveniently (?), the company that sold the dietary supplements was also on the same floor as the surgery. My friend had informed me to have about €300 to €400 on me, so when it came to paying I was able to cough up the €320 for the two months' supply of 'medical' supplements. I took my supplements and went home.

At home, I lined up the little bottles and sat down to read the diet plan. The only real food that I was allowed to eat was green salad with olive oil: no lemon juice and no vinegar. It reminded me of the vegetarian diet which eventually turned out to be a detoxification process. I didn't manage to find many foodstuffs on the diet plan he had given me, in fact – there was no food. But as it concerns the supplements, I was taking these by the handful.

After a while, my friends asked me how I was coping with the diet and if I was experiencing any problems. I told them that it was a bit stressful, but the little bottles prevented me from feeling hunger pangs. Indeed, I lost five kilos in two months. But I wasn't eating food – I was subsisting on dietary supplements. At the second appointment, he put me on a four month program and gave me four months' worth of dietary supplements at a cost of €380. Once again, I was simply consuming supplements – but very little real food. By the time of the third appointment, I had lost eleven kilos, and he put me on a six month program and gave me six months' worth of dietary supplements at a cost of €450. Naturally, I quit because I couldn't take any more without eating real food.

11 DUKAN DIET – *A failure as it concerns sustenance*
Since I couldn't get any joy from alternative dietary methods, I reverted to the classical methods. And so I embarked on the Dukan diet. This diet is based on proteins, but it is not as strict as the older protein based dietary methods.

By the end of the week, I had lost two and a half kilos, but this was accompanied by intestinal problems – something which was quite new for me.

At that time, during an outing with some friends, I met a couple who were very enthusiastic about this diet. They were in the third stage of the programme, and they had both lost a lot of weight; the man, who was fatter, had lost more kilos. At some point in the conversation, though, the man confessed that he was frightened of the pre-maintenance stage because of its long duration.

"I'm already exhausted, and I think I'm going to crack. The good thing so far has been my wife's encouragement; if it hadn't been for her, I would have quit." he said. I was in the second week – and labouring. Once again, I was on a diet that included meat, and I didn't like it. I had become involved once more in a monotonous dietary procedure which reminded me of some of those old unsuccessful dietary programmes, so – I quit.

SO WHY DO ALL DIETS FAIL?

The majority of diets promise – a lot! If someone faithfully and strictly follows a diet – weight will be lost. But in a short space of time, those lost kilos will be regained little by little. What could be to blame for this?

The fundamental underlying principles of dieting are to blame: and in particular the central principle – dieting will lead rapidly to weight loss by eating only certain foods. We've all seen book titles with wording such as the full plate …, the ultimate diet …, the metabolic effect diet …, making the cut …, the fat belly …, the Mediterranean …, and so forth.

Personally, I believe that all these books are based on faulty premises: you and I don't only want to continuously lose weight – we also want to maintain our proper body weight. We don't want to remain in a perpetually obese state that makes our lives difficult: we want a solution to our weight problems, and that is why we seek the advice of doctors and dieticians.

This, of course, presupposes a slower rate of weight loss; a more balanced diet; and, fundamentally, a proven dietary programme: such a programme will ideally have been studied for several years, and its results will have been shown to be positive as it concerns its application – as opposed to the hypothetically effective dietary programmes that appear in diet books year after year. Let's now see why, according to my experience, there are problems associated with the various diets.

1 DIETS DON'T FACTOR IN TASTE
The majority of the diets that I had followed were boring and monotonous: there was little or no variation in the flavours of the various foodstuffs in the diet. A fat person, such as me, likes to taste a variety of flavours: sweet, salty, bitter, and sour.

At some point in my diet, I was forbidden to eat legumes, fruit, and foods such as raisins and dried fruit; instead, I was put on a diet of protein based foods and vegetables, and – for what it was worth – a little 2% milk or 2% yoghurt, and a few cereals to prevent me from getting fed up with the diet. The result was that I had no choice as it concerned flavour. So, one could say that every diet results in a war against the taste buds. It seemed to me that I was only using half or less than half of my taste buds. This isn't on – my dear specialist. Find me a 'recipe' that includes all the flavours and at the same time – allows me to slim

2 DIETS IMPLEMENT STRICT PROGRAMMES

If overweight people could adhere properly to a strict dietary programme that produces quick results, those people wouldn't put on weight – and they would no longer be fat. But this model is wrong because the key factor is what the expert insinuates "Because up until now you weren't on a dietary programme, and you didn't eat the proper foods – come here and I'll sternly tell you exactly what you have to do. And you'll have to do what I tell you." It's almost as if they were being punished for not having 'performed' well.

In other words, you (the overweight person) made a mistake. This gives rise to a characteristic syndrome and associated feelings of guilt: whilst on the programme, you are in an uncomfortable state of constantly being on the defensive. You obey the experts because you need them, but as soon as the programme is completed, you revert to your old habits: this in turn necessitates you seeking the assistance of the experts again – and the whole cycle is repeated once more. Because of this, the relationship becomes stressful and problematic; indeed, this is borne out by research which proves that dieting is exceptionally stressful: throughout the period of dieting, stress hormones levels substantially increase.

3 DIETS ARE CONCERNED WITH HOW MUCH YOU EAT – NOT WHY YOU EAT

All nutritional models stress the quantitative mistakes associated with eating, that is: it all centres on how many calories we should be consuming. Although this is also a factor, a more important factor is the reason that we eat as much as we do. Do we need to eat such amounts? Are we really hungry? And the answer is that in actual fact – we are not hungry.

Specialists pass over the question of 'Why do we eat?' The psychology and self-esteem of those who want to diet is not something that is uppermost in their minds: some probably consider it, but as a secondary matter. Thus, most of the time, overweight people can't focus on the objective of slimming; they can't keep alive the motivation to slim, and consequently they return to their old habits because here they feel secure, dependent on their food, and above all – satisfaction.

The dietary model that is currently in force is based on a 'family' model where the man goes to his 'dad specialist' and the woman goes to her 'mum specialist' and they give them – the successful recipe for losing weight. The overweight person becomes trapped in this relationship: remaining psychologically in the role of the child: and in order not disappoint 'mum' or 'dad' – they do what they are told. In this way, the overweight person withdraws into himself again and once more puts on weight. Consequently, a vicious circle is perpetuated: psychological vacuum – food – success – overweight – guilt – psychological vacuum – food – success – overweight – guilt – …

4 DIETS PROMISE RAPID RESULTS

Slimming 'recipes' promise us rapid, easy, and simple solutions: diets in five minutes or in five steps – simple diets. In actual fact, such diets don't exist. In order to lose weight, you have to spend time on yourself, your diet, and you will have to discover which recipes are suitable for you. Those who have managed to lose weight and maintain their proper body weight are often those people who have been on suitable dietary programmes for many years. Taking myself as an example, for the past few years – I have weighed about 127 kilos. If I am to achieve my proper body weight, I will have to lose fifty-five kilos. Now, I ask you: "Is it really possible to rapidly lose this number of kilos?"

5 DIETS SET UNREALISTIC TARGETS

Almost all diets are unrealistic. They promise you results if you adhere to them properly; they also promise you will lose lots of weight in the space of a few weeks or months. But not a single diet will advise you to set a target of losing only half a kilo a month and thereby avoid causing shock to your body by not making significant changes to your daily routine. In this way, you will have lost six kilos in the first year; twelve kilos by the end of the second year; and eighteen kilos by the end of the third year. Besides, who really believes that body weight which has been accumulating for years can possibly be lost in three to four months? No logical person would believe this.

That's why you should set realistic targets. In this way, you can substitute healthy foods for bad foods – and you will gain health.

6 DIETS MAINTAIN THE OLD HABITS

Overweight people know within them where the mistake is. After sometime, they understand that changes need to be made: but they either don't know how to make those changes or they dare not make them alone, so they consult books and specialists – and that's where they get lost. The problem gets 'recycled' and they become disappointed: what are needed are new habits. Someone should tell them that by creating new habits, the old ones will be eliminated, and they will be able to get out of the impasse they find themselves in. But does anyone ever do it? No, of course. A new habit does not mean starting a new dietary programme; nor does it mean pressuring oneself to lose weight on such a programme: it means changing what you used to do in the morning, in the afternoon, and in the evening. A new habit means not associating food with the various things happening in your personal or professional life; it means finding daily motivation; it means thinking positively about yourself and keeping a diary. From new habits, a new you will emerge: since the new you is the new daily routine which is determined by you. Unfortunately, not a single specialist bothers with this matter.

7 DIETS CREATE MYTHS ABOUT SUPERFOODS

Every year, specialists discover new foodstuffs with hidden therapeutic ingredients, and new nutritional combinations for slimming. Does eating grapefruits really contribute to weight loss? Do egg white, asparagus, green tea, and apple vinegar have dietary value? Where do the myths stop and the truth begin? It is on such myths that a whole industry has sprung up for the production of low calorie drinks, natural products, and confectionery. Researchers, however, take another view: they stress that we should not be misled because there are no such things as – miracle foods. The idea that some discovery or new method of food combination will immediately alter your weight or your health problem(s) – is, more often than not, the result of bad information. Neither your health nor your weight can be immediately influenced for the better.

It should also be noted that the exclusion of certain foodstuffs from a diet for the purpose of weight loss may deprive the brain of valuable nutrients, and it also increases the risk of prematurely terminating the diet.

8 DIETS SERVE THE IDEAL

Living a high lifestyle can be very exciting, but when you have to do with ordinary people – the demands have to be adjusted accordingly. We expect film stars to be beautiful, and athletes to have well-proportioned bodies, and we all admire them for these qualities. But if you see them after they have retired from acting and sports, their physical appearance is truly something to be pitied: aged faces, sagging breasts, and legs that are so misshaped that they cannot fail to elicit either sorrow or laughter. In contrast to the stars and the athletes, the ordinary man in the street just wants to lose weight for reasons of health: excess weight causes problems. This is a fundamental factor that a specialist should take into consideration, and if an overweight person is rambling on about wanting to look beautiful, the specialist should quickly bring the overweight person back down to earth: images of the ideal body must be put aside, and the design of the dietary programme should be aimed at reducing weight. For example, no specialist, prior to prescribing a dietary programme, has ever asked me how much weight I would like to lose or I believe I could lose. Well, if I were to say five kilos in one year, I would be thrown out. My ideal weight was always determined on the basis of my height and actual body weight. And achieving the ideal weight was the ultimate goal with one 'small' proviso – I had to lose tens of kilos, and, of course, I didn't succeed in doing that. Thus, I continued to gain and lose weight in a vicious circle: even after going on a new dietary programme. If someone had said to me that I have to lose ONLY five kilos a year, it's certain that I would have got rid of a lot of weight forever. Unfortunately, the whole concept of dieting rests on the notion of the ideal: the ideal weight, the ideal body, and the ideal man. And in reality – this does not exist, but this doesn't obstruct the appearance of 'prejudice'.

9 THEY DON'T TELL YOU THAT YOU'LL HAVE TO DIET FOR THE REST OF YOUR LIFE

In the USA, 80% of girls say they have been on some sort of a diet programme by the time they are ten. (Sandra Aamodt is a neuroscientist and science writer: see talk at TEDGlobal 2013.) Neither these children nor I were told (although I had started dieting at an older age) that when you start a diet – you never stop. For the whole of your life you will have to follow a dietary regime; otherwise, you will regain those lost kilos. Personally speaking, if I were to embark on a diet and my dietician were to inform me that I would have to survive on his prescribed diet for the rest of my life – I would stop the diet and change dietician.

I think this is something that all obese people would do – leading, eventually, to the demise of dietetics. It is, however, a truth that should be stated clearly from the beginning – dieting is for life.

I GAVE UP ON THE SPECIALISTS & RECOVERED MY HEALTH

I quit seeing specialists; I got my health back and discovered a big truth.

After so many fruitless (no pun intended) diets, I started thinking about giving up trying to lose weight: I was in a very negative frame of mind. I wanted to reset the 'speedometer' and independently seek out the mistakes and the causes that were preventing me from losing weight. I had gone on quite a few diets; I had read a lot of health books; and because of my work, I kept abreast of the latest news and research concerned with medical matters.

I started off by keeping a very detailed log. I was certain that if I recorded everything I ate, I would get a true picture of my diet: I would be able to monitor how many times I ate, what I ate, and what my eating habits were. In the log, each foodstuff was accompanied by a description of its principal nutritional content, e.g. protein, carbohydrate, and so forth. I knew, from research, that all those who had managed to lose a lot of weight over many years had managed to do it alone. So, I designed my own dietary programme with those foods (in reasonable amounts) that I enjoyed. Relieved from the anxiety of having to think about whether I would lose weight; if I would lose weight; how much weight I would lose; and how long it would take to lose weight - I followed my diet to the letter. I had no problem during the day, but in the evening I would surrender to a craving for something sweet. When I was at home, I would open the fridge and all the cupboards in search of anything sweet which if found – I would gobble up. Whenever I was out, I would walk into the first patisserie that I saw. I felt as helpless as an alcoholic: it didn't matter what it was as long as it had a sweet flavour. I didn't care if it was black chocolate, white chocolate, cake, jam, doughnuts, or ice cream. My problem was so serious that I couldn't control it.

At that time, I was also reading books about medicine in ancient Greece. In "On the Nature of Man" (volume 4 in the Hippocratic collection) reference is made to the equilibrium of the four humours (this matter is also dealt with in Galen's "On the Humours"). According to these ancients, balance and health depend on the equilibrium of the four humours which reside in the human body: the predominance of any one humour results in disequilibrium and illness. At this point, my mind registered that because of this we are in a state of disequilibrium in respect of our diets. Indeed, Alcmaeon refers to the equality of forces: including the bitter and the sweet forces. (Aetios, V 30, 1)

The next day on my way home from work, I again felt a craving for something sweet, so I bought a kantaifi with lashings of syrup. When I got home, I sat down at the table to enjoy my oriental sweet and at the same time I took something to read out of my bag. I only managed to swallow the first mouthful because by the second mouthful I had lost my appetite – why? I was reading a research article concerning the consumer's dependency on sugar: the conclusions were shocking. According to the article, we react to sugar addiction in the same way as a drug addict reacts to drugs or an alcoholic to alcohol; this was exactly what I was experiencing, and I could not control myself: a nutritional imbalance and an addiction to sweet flavours, viz. – sugar. My mind was preoccupied with these two things for days.

Thus, at some point, I looked in my log again and beginning from the first day I started to characterize the flavours of all the foods I had eaten, for example: potato – sweet, meat – sweet, spaghetti – sweet, chocolate – sweet, and so on. I got a new shock when I saw that 90% of my diet – which I thought was healthy – consisted of sweet and salty flavours: I hadn't been eating any bitter tasting foods and very few sour ones. I kept on looking and looking at my log. Afterwards, I started looking for what scientific material was available on the subject, and I was left utterly gobsmacked. I discovered that a lot of researches arrived at a very important truth, viz. discovery, but this is not communicated to people. Eureka! I dived in at the deep end and started to research.

CHAPTER 2
THE PROBLEM

There are three contributory factors that make people fat: first, the person that gave birth to you feeds you with whatever they have been accustomed to eating (predominantly sweet and salty tasting foods) and in doing so they transfer their bad nutritional habits to you; second, once the child reaches adolescence, the food industry is allowed, either actively or passively, to take over the individual's diet – thereby giving it 'identity' and 'style'. Here, again, we are primarily confined to either sweet tasting or salty tasting foods.

Third, the portions we eat are for giants and not for people whose daily lives are for a large part of the day confined in an office, or sitting behind a desk, or behind the steering wheel of a car. Initially, we will have to understand the problem of obesity before we can combat it: the scientific community recognizes the problem, and some courageous scientists speak out and reveal it. Let's now look at the problem step by step.

DON'T 'KILL' YOUR CHILD WITH THE WRONG FLAVOURS

It sounds crazy, but it's absolutely true: mothers are 'killing' their children with the food they feed them. While in the womb, the child becomes accustomed to recognizing the various flavours, and by the time the child is conceived the damage has already been done. From a logically point of view, sentimentality and scientific research aside, the child is blameless since it is ignorant of the world it is brought into. We teach our children what to eat, how to eat, and when to eat. The 'crime' of bad nutrition that leads to obesity starts and ends with us. Mothers fail to accustom their children to foods containing all of the four flavours because they themselves do not eat such foods. Thus, a child who has become accustomed to, say, sweet flavoured foods, will always have a craving for sweet flavours. Scientific research supports the view that preferences for various flavours start with the mother because the embryo is exposed to and influenced by its mother's preferences.

Prenatally, the mother's diet nourishes the foetus via the amniotic fluid and maternal blood; postnatal, the foetus is nourished by the mother's maternal milk. In fact, newborn children's sense of taste is the most important and most developed of all the senses. This has been demonstrated experimentally by the Centre for the Science of Taste in Dijon: experts conducted experiments on twenty-four babies (whose mothers had eaten anise flavoured biscuits in the ten day period prior to birth) several hours after birth and four days later. It was found that these babies recognized and enjoyed the taste of anise.

Another study showed that when mothers drank carrot juice regularly during pregnancy or while breastfeeding, infants exhibited fewer negative facial expressions when tasting carrot flavoured cereals compared with plain cereals.

Additionally, those embryos that were prenatally exposed to carrots gave their mothers the impression that they enjoyed carrot flavoured cereals more than plain cereals. (*See ref. 1*)

It is therefore indisputable that the mother influences the food choices of her offspring. While the facts in support of this are still few in number, it is certain that newborn children recognize different flavours and react to them differently even before they have been exposed to them: and these initial taste reactions relate to sweet, bitter, and sour flavours. As it concerns the perception of a salty flavour: it appears to develop from the age of six months. This is why the mother should follow a balanced diet, which is as 'natural' as possible and contains all the flavours (*See ref. 2*)

The eating habits developed during the foetal stage, the period of breastfeeding, and the early years of growth follow the child throughout its life, and they are difficult to change.

"Dietary patterns are formed during the period that spans the inception of life to the end of childhood, but from the moment they are formed: they are very difficult to change even when the child has grown up. Think about how difficult it would be to change the things that you like to eat as an adult. You could change them, but it would be really difficult: at the end of the day, you'll be back at square one – eating the same old foods." (*See ref. 3*)

This means that parents who incorrectly feed their children with foods containing only two flavours (sweet and salty), and processed foods are laying the foundations for their future obesity.

This confirms the research carried out by the Food Plus research centre of the University of Adelaide in South Australia which found that exposure to "a high calorie diet deficient in nutrients (junk food) makes children prefer the same high calorie foods." When researchers studied mice, they found that exposure to such foods during intra-uterine life, and during lactation led to the creation of a reward circuit in the brain which, though, was found to be less sensitive than expected.

It is certain that sweet flavours have an analgesic effect on babies and children since they cry less when they have something sweet in their mouths. And as the child grows up, it connects sweet flavours with pleasant memories: a friendly gathering at home, a children's party, and a children's birthday with its biscuits, cakes, and jellies. In a few words, the child forms a positive link between sweet flavours and enjoyable activities such as holidays, celebrations, receiving good news, smiling, and other happy occasions.

But could you have a children's party with foods such as broccoli, arugula (rocket), lettuce, apples and other fruit? It would certainly be a novel idea. But celebrations and parties with sweet tasting foods could become the exception in a balanced diet for children – and even for adults – instead of the continuing daily unbalanced diet.

Moreover, if the parents have a humdrum diet (only with sweet and salty flavours) consisting of processed foods, and foods tainted with pesticides, insecticides, and other chemical compounds – this creates a problem for the foetus. These compounds produce oestrogen mimetic effects which disturb hormone levels: primarily in males. It should be noted that oestrogen is a female hormone.

Even if parents nourish themselves with 'rubbish' food, there is still the possibility that the child may exhibit symptoms of nutritional neophobia; viz. the child develops a fear of trying new foodstuffs, and flavours. The phenomenon occurs mainly between the ages of two and six and the problem is best dealt with by actively co-operating with the child rather than simply dismissing the problem. According to research, up to ten repeated exposures are required before a child becomes accustomed to a new food. Doctors are of the opinion that putting the novel food – the new flavour – in a small amount next to the food that the child is already accustomed to eating will slowly reduce the child's negative reaction to the former: the same result can be achieved when the child sees the parent(s) experimenting with new foods and new flavours.

It is certain that a liking for eating fruit and vegetables should be developed by the time the child has reached the age of twelve months; otherwise, as the child grows up – it will avoid these foods.

In France, for instance, parents consider it their duty to teach their children that each food has its own nutritional value and that we should not reject any foods. The rule is that although children do not have to eat it all, it is necessary to try it. (*See ref. 4*)

As it concerns the need to inform parents about the effects of an early balanced diet on children's health, this has been established by another research programme, which was conducted in eleven countries.

According to the data, health professionals are of the opinion that parents don't appreciate the beneficial value that a balanced diet has for the nutritional future of their children.

The child's exposure to all flavours determines its dietary habits in adulthood; above all, it is the key to eating fruits and vegetables.

Nowadays, with children consuming so many sweet and salty (savoury) flavoured foods, this is having unpleasant effects on their bodies. For example, youngsters who eat fast food, sweets, and drink fizzy drinks have arteries like an old man's. The problem is caused by glycotoxins ('burned' proteins): dangerous toxic substances that are created during the thermal processing of foods and which prevent the body cells from being renewed. These substances accumulate over time; they weaken the immune system and they oxidize the body cells.

They are also associated with chronic diseases such as obesity – here we go again; there it is confronting us once more – dementia, diabetes, atherosclerosis, hypertension, heart disease, kidney disease, arthritis, osteoporosis, dermal and epidermal aging, periodontal diseases, and so on.

And they are found in many highly processed snacks, refined foods (powdered milk and powdered eggs), and pre-prepared frozen meals that can be cooked in microwave ovens because these contain glycotoxins even before cooking. Additionally, glycotoxins are also created by the use of 'bad' methods of cooking: such as frying and barbecuing.

Moreover, girls who consume more than a normal amount of sugary drinks have menstruate earlier according to a study published in the journal "Human Reproduction".

The 'antidote' for all of this is to eat a variety of healthy foods from an early age coupled with living in a better environment. (*See ref. 5*)

SUPERMARKETS HAVE BECOME PATISSERIES

When you shop at a supermarket, do you ever question whether you are actually in a supermarket? Well, you aren't in a supermarket – you are in a patisserie with supermarket shop signs on the outside. You are effectively in a patisserie because the dominant food flavour is sweet: salty (savoury) flavoured foods come second. Can you recall any bitter tasting food you recently saw on a supermarket shelf and then purchased? It might be hard for you to remember because most of the shelves are taken up with sauces, soups, chocolate biscuits, sweets, bread, desserts, soft drinks, ice cream, snacks, flour, pasta, sausages, dairy products, processed frozen foods, jams, marmalades, and many other sweet flavoured products which are prominent on the shelves of a supermarket. The sweet flavour – that is sugar – goes under many different names that we are not aware of when shopping sugar containing foodstuffs. It often appears on the labels of packaged foods as one of the following names: lactose, glucose, dextrose, malt extract, castor sugar, invert sugar, isoglucose, brown sugar, lactose, maltose, maltodextrin, molasses, agave nectar, sucrose, glucose syrup, syrup or cane juice, brown sugar syrup, rice syrup, fructose corn syrup, modified starch, and fructose. At the present, sugar is contained in 75% of all packaged products purchased in the USA: the average American consumes between 125 to 200 grams of sugar per day! (*See ref. 6*)

And if what is on the supermarket shelves is not sweet, then it is salty. These are the nutritional choices in our cities that the food industry has provided us with: choices which addict us to sickly flavoured foods which fatten us and cause us health problems. And almost all research confirms that they contribute and cause illnesses in addition to obesity, for example: hypertension, diabetes, heart problems, and cancer – exactly those illnesses that people die from nowadays. The over consumption of such foods is currently part of the worldwide diet: it is the diet of two flavours.

And why are the supermarket shelves full of foodstuffs with these two flavours? Because the food industry derives its strength from these two flavours: it knows that they make you feel happy, and the happier you feel the more addicted you become – so you get hooked to the foodstuffs that satisfy your craving for these flavours. It is worth noting that the average number of products sold in a supermarket in 1977 was 10,000; whereas now, it exceeds 30,000 which, of course, also include non-food products. There are now literally thousands of products to caress the palate and add calories to the consumer's diet.

But how did we get to this state? We got to this state for several reasons that can be traced back to the 70s: consumers were bombarded with ads for high calorie ready meals with high fat content, and drinks with high sugar content; vending machines for beverages and sweets sprouted up everywhere; fast food outlets became a permanent feature of shopping malls; and we started drastically reducing the use of our hands for various tasks and our feet for walking.

Another reason was that women came into the labour market at that time: this presented a new buying force which was catered for by the appearance of mass produced tasty, cheap ready-made foods: prepared with sugar, salt, and fat – and rich in calories.

And how does a foodstuff become tasty? Snacking is 'criminalized', but it is those chemicals that also produce a pleasant sensation in alcoholic drinks, chewing gum, sweets that enhance the appearance of mushrooms, roots, bulbs, tubers, nuts, and which are also used for spicing red meats, poultry, game, and fish.

Acids are also employed for many purposes in the food industry. They are used for improving the raw materials used in the confectionery industry, and in foodstuffs such as canned fruit and vegetables, fruit juices, marmalades and jams, pasta foods, and chocolates. They are used for improving food colouring in foodstuffs such as jellies, mustards, instant soups, soft drinks, margarine, oil, butter, and cheese. They are also used as additives for making foodstuffs softer or crunchier. Finally, additive enzymes and seasonings are used in bread, diet products, and buns. The catalogue of uses is almost endless. According to scientists researching in taste: a food can have the flavour of a particular fruit without being that fruit. In other words, the apple taste, say, used as an ingredient in a foodstuff may not have been extracted from real apples, but is merely an artificially produced flavour.

YOU AREN'T EATING FOOD – YOU ARE TAKING YOUR DRUGS

It could be said that over the last few decades, you haven't been eating your food, but – taking you drugs. A lot of research has been done which shows the addictive effects of salty (savoury) and sweet flavours on the human brain: researchers accept the view that once someone becomes addicted, they are unable to control the amount of food they eat because addictive food makes someone happy, and redefines the person's relationship with their food – thereby creating new eating habits. Additionally, sweet flavours further stimulate appetite. Unfortunately, no dietary programme involves itself with this issue which is at the heart of the problem of obesity. So what does research tell us? It tell us that the daily consumption of sugar causes neurochemical changes in the brain which resemble those produced in the brain of someone who takes drugs such as cocaine, morphine, and heroin, or who takes nicotine by smoking. Some research shows that the effect is even stronger than that of hard drugs.

Indeed, the lack of sweet flavours manifests itself in the form of anxiety, tremors, depression, low spirits, fatigue, headaches, and quivers. Does this all sound familiar? Furthermore, addiction and deprivation effects equally apply to salty flavours.

Many who managed to wean themselves off drugs became addicted to sweet flavours and subsequently became obese. From the moment they quits drugs, the brain asks for other rewards such as chocolate, biscuits, and anything that has sugar: their addiction is transferred to something else. They say "No" to cocaine, but "Yes" to sugar. (*See ref. 7*)

Interestingly, in the Big Book of Alcoholics Anonymous – where the twelve steps to detox are set out – it is shown that those who are in recovery can have access to sugary foods. Succinctly, it is sugar and not fat that causes in us a mania for food. (*See ref. 8*)

It is worth noting that American scientists, in an article entitled "The toxic truth about sugar" which was published in the well-known scientific journal 'Nature', actually proposed that sugar should be taxed. They argued that sugar should be subject to excise duty similar to that put on alcohol and tobacco because it is addictive and harmful to the body.

Indeed, very tasty foods – the kind served in fast food outlets and restaurant chains – change the chemistry of the brain thereby triggering a neurological response that stimulates people to eat more food – even when they are not hungry. (*See ref. 9*)

One more reason that obese people eat more is because obesity alters the intensity pf the flavour. Studies have shown that obese people constantly seek sweet and generally richly flavoured foods because they cannot perceive these flavours to same degree as they are perceived by thinner people.

Another study published on the online version 'Open Heart' contends that sugar is worse than salt as an agent for increasing blood pressure. Specifically, the researchers argue that those who use more than 74 grams of corn syrup, with a high fructose content (a sweetener used in highly processed foods such as soft drinks) have a 30% increased risk of developing hypertension.

Particularly worrying is the case of adolescents who consume too many processed sugars – often 16 times over the recommended limit. The report was cosigned by Dr. James di Nikolantonio (an expert in cardiovascular health) of Cardiology Institute St. Luke together with Dr. Sean Shi Luka of the Albert Einstein Medical School of New York. (Dr James DiNicolantonio, at the Saint Luke's Mid America Heart Institute, published the paper, with Dr Sean C Lucan, of the Albert Einstein College of Medicine in New York.)

Both sugar and meat 'nourish' cancer. Two principal characteristics of the tumor cell metabolism are an increased needs for glucose (they require 10 to 50 times more glucose relative to healthy cells) and methionine (an amino acid found in animal proteins which has a high intake especially in the consumption of meat).

Cravings for sweets, refined carbohydrates, and meat eating are associated with weight gain and the deposition of fat in the abdomen (abdominal obesity). This situation leads to metabolic, inflammatory, and oxidative stress products which promote the emergence and worsening of cancer. (*See ref. 10*)

In another study it was determined that the sugar molecule named Neu5Gc, which is located in beef, pork, and lamb, is responsible for the appearance of cancer: this molecule is present in the bodies of all mammals – except for humans. Consequently, when you eat red meat, your body sees the Neu5Gc molecule as a foreign substance thus causing the immune system to attack it. This leads to inflammation of the body, which can over time develop into a tumor. The same situation can occur when people consume whole milk, cheeses, and fish eggs.

The lead researcher of the University of California, Dr. Varki, does not recommend the elimination of red meat from our eating habits. According to Dr. Varki: "The controlled consumption of meat is a source of nutrition for humans. Over consumption, however, can lead to the emergence of various forms of cancer." (*See ref.11*)

Scientists have been telling us for the last fifty years that worldwide consumption of sugar thus has tripled: exacerbating obesity and other diseases. In 2003 the WHO (World Health Organization) issued a recommendation that the daily intake of sugar should not exceed more than 10% of the daily number of calories. Of course, nothing happened since in many Western countries a diet based on sweet flavours is a "national dish": with the percentage daily intake of sugar reaching up to 25% of daily calorie intake.

So in 2014, the WHO came back with a recommendation that the daily consumption of sugar should be set at the lower limit of not more than 5%. But that's crazy! People didn't comply with the 10% limit and now they have to get it down to a 5% threshold?

A lot of research has been carried out on the effects of salt and sugar by some of the best universities in the world. The conclusions included the following findings: although their consumption causes pleasant sensations, it also results in long-lasting changes to the brain; sugary substances can suppress leptin – the hormone which controls hunger and feelings of satiety; foods loaded with sugar and salt which are specifically made to appeal to consumers trigger overeating in people predisposed to addiction; processed foods rich in sugar illuminate the same areas of the brain that are activated when taking hard drugs.

Thus, the addiction to fattening foods could explain why weight loss is difficult and why those who follow a diet fail to strictly follow it. Well, after all this – are you still trying to find out why you are putting on weight?

From an evolutionary point of view, however, our ancestors ate sugar only for a few months of the year: when eating seasonal fruit or honey. They didn't have access to the many different forms of sugar throughout the whole year, which is something that we have nowadays.

British research, undertaken at the university of Dundee and UCL, warns us that a lot of patients who take the maximum daily dosage of various common medicines (such as painkillers, aspirins, and cough medicines) unwittingly risk exceeding the daily recommended limit for salt intake: even though they may be regulating their diet in order not to exceed their daily salt intake.

These preparations (mainly carbonated preparations, e.g. carbonated soluble tablets) contain sodium salts in order to improve their solubility and subsequent absorption by the body. Taking other risk factors into account (such as weight, smoking, alcohol, and patient history), the researchers concluded that patients who took medicines containing sodium salts had, on average, a 16% increased risk of heart attack, stroke, or death from cardiovascular disease compared with those patients taking similar medicines, but without sodium salts. They were also seven times more likely to develop hypertension, and the risk of death – irrespective of the cause – was, on average, 28% higher.

THE SIZE OF YOUR PLATE AND THE FLAVOUR
OF YOUR FOOD IS FATTENING

The third factor that has contributed to the increase in obesity is big portions: this is because the food packaging is labelled with catchy words such as 'giant' and 'family' in order to more easily entice shoppers to buy. And sold at promotional prices, these foods are more easily consumed by tired households. In fact, the sales of these foods have been growing over the decades – 'pumping' us up with more and more calories.

Now that our life has become easier and more sedentary – so we need fewer calories – portions have become larger and more addictive. They have actually increased by 35%!

According to a survey by the University of North Carolina, the average daily calorie intake from the 1970s until now has increased from 1,803 calories to 2,374. Indeed, in the last decade, the average daily calorie intake has increased by an additional 229 calories.

Nowadays, the average daily portion has increased by 800 calories. Yes, you read that correctly – 800 calories. 800 calories of ever more fattening food for a daily routine that requires little physical exertion or manual work. But someone should have explained to you that if you eat normal portions with all the flavours, you shouldn't have any problems. And what are normal portions? Definitely not those portions that come on 30 cm diameter plates. The following study will clearly show you the effect of big portions. Cornell University (USA) conducted a study on a group of children to see the effect of big portions. Children who had been given large bowls requested 87% more milk and cereals compared with those who had been given smaller bowls and it was found, as expected, that the large bowl children consumed more calories: in fact, they consumed

52% more calories in total. Subsequently, the researchers suggested that plates should not exceed a diameter of 25 cm: since the smaller plate is a truer measure of how much you eat.

References

1. http://www.ncbi.nlm.nih.gov/pubmed/11389286 .
2. Professor Benoist Schaal center of State for Science of Taste in Dijon (CNRS-University of Burgundy).
3. New York Times. Wartman K. Bad Eating Habits Start in the Womb.
    http://www.nytimes.com/2013/12/02/opinion/bad-eating-habits-start-in-the-womb.html?pagewanted=all.
4. Druckerman P. (2012) French Children Don't Throw Food. Great Britain: Dobleday.
5. Polyxena Nikolopoulou-Stamatis, Professor of Athens Medical School.
6. http://www.nytimes.com/2014/12/23/opinion/sugar-season-its-everywhere-and-addictive.html?_r=0 .
7. Dr. Pamela Peeke, assistant professor of medicine at the University of Maryland and author of "The Hunger Fix."
8. http://www.ncbi.nlm.nih.gov/pubmed/24132980 .
9. Kessler D. A. (2010) The End of Overeating. Great Britain: Penguin. (Dr. Kessler was a former representative of the USA Food and Drug Administration – FDA).
10. Despina Komnenos, physician, nutritionist, and scientific advisor to the Institute of Applied Biosciences at the Greek National Centre for Research and Technological Development.
11. http://www.pnas.org/content/100/21/12045.full?sid=5db45e72-ac2d-42fb-bbf9-df4f1b1c-58bc .

CHAPTER 3
THE SOLUTION

SOUR & BITTER FLAVOURS ARE THERAPEUTIC

Thinking back to my childhood days, I remember when we were sat around the table for meals with my family or other relatives, there were foods whose flavours weren't particularly 'child friendly': sour and bitter flavours which we didn't like since novel foods with appealing sweet flavours had now made their appearance on the table.

Our parents and grandparents, who had been brought up on bitter and sour fla-voured foods, considered these novel foods a little bit strange – they just couldn't seem to get used to them. But like all children, whenever faced with the choice of a bottle of sweet tasting fizzy orangeade or a glass of natural orange juice, we always chose the fizzy drink. So in order to encourage us to drink natural fruit juices, my mother used to put a little sugar in it. Apart from natural orange juice, we also had homemade lemonade, which was much worse – it was really bitter. But the worst of all were – the herbal drinks. The adults drank them daily with unadulterated pleasure while for us: just their odour was enough to make our stomachs turn. Indeed, all the children of my generation associated bitter and sour flavours with some illness or other. And why was that? Because when we were ill with typical children's illnesses, they used to give us bitter herbal teas to drink; unfortunately, the doctor's cough medicine was equally bitter.

Now, I'd like to ask you. "When was the last time that you ate something bitter? How many times a day or a week do you eat anything bitter? For the majority of people in the Western world, the answer to the latter question will be: "Rarely". Forty to fifty years ago, people were closer to nature, and they derive more of their knowledge of foods and diet from it: they ate bitter flavoured wild fruits and wild greens during the four seasons of the year – because, you see, nature doesn't produce sugary 'products'.

Today, bitter flavours have disappeared because our diet is determined by the food industry, supermarkets, advertisements, experts, and the unrealistic 'plastic bodies' of well-known personalities.

Even vegetables are debittered before they are put on the market; in contrast, sugar and sweeteners are added to fruit juices, and some wines are scientifically treated in order to reduce their bitterness. In foods, phytonutrients are of the utmost importance: taste is of secondary importance; however, when it comes to bitter tasting foods, the converse applies: now taste predominates (in order to sweeten it), and phytonutrients play a secondary role.

In this way, the rich natural 'arsenal' of compounds that bitter foods possess is lost: these compounds, which have antioxidant activity, also constitute a shield against diseases.

Who has not heard or has not read that a diet rich in green leafy vegetables and cruciferous vegetables protects humans from heart disease, hypertension, diabetes, and cancer? This is something that everyone probably knows.

Apart from being rich in vitamins, minerals and fiber, research has shown that bitter and sour tasting substances are beneficial for the human body: they strengthen and detoxify the liver and by doing so, the liver doesn't have to work excessively in order to produce insulin; they are fortifying and bring about physical wellbeing; they improve metabolism and in this way cholesterol levels can be lowered; they assist in weight loss; and they help with digestion so that more nutrients to be absorbed.

Although there is knowledge about such foods, it is not applied in our daily lives. Bitter flavoured foods are an important dietary part of those populations having high longevity: in those populations which subsist on traditional diets, bitter flavoured foods are found in the forms of wild greens, fruit, and herbal drinks.

Even nowadays, in the rural areas of Greece it is considered a pleasure to collect wild herbs and fruits that flourish in spring, autumn and winter. In many regions, salads are made with a variety of foods, for example: common chicory (*Cichori-*

um intybus), common dandelions (*Taraxacum officinale*), wild artichokes (*Cynara cardunculus*), cultivated artichokes (*Cynara scolymus L.*), edible Muscari (*Muscari comosum*), purslane (*Portulaca oleracea*), nettles (*Urtica dioica*), Shepherd's needle (*Scandix pectin veneris L.*), prickly goldenfleece (*Urospermum picroides*), and many others – all of which are bitter flavoured.

Additionally, for decades now, the use of various herbs has been a characteristic of Greek cooking. Some of the more common herbs used are as follows: oregano (*origanum onites*), basil (*ocimum basilicum L.*), marjoram (*origanum majorana*), thyme (*thymus sibthorpii benth.*), peppermint (*mentha*), rosemary (*rosmarinus officinalis*), laurel (*laurus nobilis L.*), and sage (*salvia officinalis*).

Diets in which wild greens and aromatic herbs are added to our food endow us with health and longevity because, according to many studies, wild greens and aromatic herbs have a high biological value (BV). However, apart from their use in cooking, bitter flavoured substances are also employed in medicine.

From the time of Homer, herbs have been described for curing diseases: ancient Greek texts listed dozens drugs which were made from roots, bark, flowers, stems, fruits, seeds, oils, and resins. In order to become medicines, they underwent relatively simple treatments, for example: pulping, drying, powdering, boiling (in water or wine) or mixing with other substances (e.g. honey or vinegar). Hippocrates, the father of medicine, recorded dozens of herbs whose use was known for their healing properties: the great pharmacologist Dioscorides and later on the other great physician Galen continued the work of recording such herbs. Indeed, many of these plant substances have been enriched in laboratories and are now well known medicines.

Greek flora provides us with therapeutic drinks and herbs: these have a high nutritional value and a dual function: they serve both as foods and medicines, and they contribute through detoxification (and other functions) in combating many disorders; they also balance the body. Indeed, research and the decades of experience in Greece have shown that the frequent intake of tisanes (e.g. concoctions made from dittany, siderite, marjoram, mint, and pennyroyal) promotes optimal health and well-being in modern man. (*See ref. 1*)

The flora of Greece is the third richest in the world with hundreds of herbs and plants that grow only in Greece: 15.6% of the plant species found in Greece are Greek endemics, i.e., they are not found anywhere else in the world. (*See ref. 2*) In fact, Europe has the highest biodiversity per unit area.

Furthermore, these herbs are rich in active substances, and a lot of them react positively against cancer, obesity, hypertension, Alzheimer's disease, heart problems, and diabetes. They also fortify the immune system; they assist in detoxification; and, they have a positive effect on the kidneys. Incidentally, all these herbs have a taste ranging from mild to very bitter. Could this be just coincidence?

And by 'active substances' we don't mean that they only cure one disease or act on a single protein target; but rather, they exhibit multifaceted therapeutic effects: thereby targeting numerous protein targets in the human body; this is not surprising since each herb can contain anything from several dozen to hundreds of active substances. This is the touchstone of modern pharmaceutical science in the field of cancer treatment: namely, the ideal combination of substances that produces a multi-targeted action. In fact, that is something that nature generously provides us with in the form of medicinal plants – and without the side effects of synthetic medicines. (*See ref. 3*)

Among the medicinal plants, whose usefulness has been demonstrated in the battle against cancer, some of the other plants that should also be included are the following: blackberries, raspberries, blueberries, cranberries, strawberries, coriander, parsley, onion, garlic, leek, olive leaf juice, nettle leaf juice, saffron, sage, rosemary, thistle, squirting cucumber, rock rose, and burdock. Once again, all these plants have either a taste ranging from mild to very sour or a bitter taste. Could this be just coincidence, again?

The anti-cancer activity of medicinal plants used in herbal medicine is many times more potent than the various standard chemotherapeutic medicines, which do not occur naturally. In phytotherapy, an illness is viewed as nothing more than an imbalance in the human body: the objective is to help the body to develop the self-healing mechanisms that it already possesses. But caution should be exercised when using medicinal herbs: on the one hand, they do not cure all diseases; and on the other hand, if you thoughtlessly use them without consulting a doctor, you may get undesired results. (*See ref. 3*)

So, before resorting to herbs, don't forget to consult your doctor. Let's now look at a few herbs that are consumed daily in the various regions of Greece where the inhabitants are blessed with longevity.

GREEK MOUNTAIN TEA ACTS AGAINST
ALTZHEIMER'S DISEASE

Professor Pahnke is a professor of neurology and director of the Research Center for Neurological Diseases at the University of Magdeburg in Germany. His study of the beneficial effects of mountain tea is well worth noting.

"For the last seven years, we have been experimenting with 150 plants and herbs from around the world, including China, Thailand, and Indonesia," recounts Professor Dr. Dr. Jens Pahnke to the Greek newspaper 'Kathimerini'. The twenty-strong scientific team analyzed the ingredients of plants and tested them on guinea pigs – but no significant results were obtained.

"From our research on the Internet, we learned about the properties of the Greek herb, ironwort (Genus: *Sideritis*), and decided to order it in 2010. We had the best results!" he adds. Specifically, when given to rats for twenty-five days, it reduced brain damage by approximately 80%; the next 'best' result was achieved by using thiethylperazin, which reduced brain damage by 70%. The thirty-eight year old professor, who annually treats 1,500 patients from around the world, also tested the properties of mountain tea on humans. "Drinking tea daily for six months, the disease reverted to the level it was nine months earlier and after that it significantly stabilized," he explains. "I had a patient who had a problem with memory and orientation, and he had reached a point where he could not even go to the toilet on his own. I gave him tea for two months and now he has improved to such an extent that he is preparing with a friend to go on holiday – in the Alps," he stresses.

For the time being, the doctor recommends drinking several cups of cold or hot tea a day. It is, moreover, well known that the earlier one takes preventive measures against the onset of Alzheimer's disease the better it will be for the individual. "Usually, you can reach the point of not remembering how to go home before you realize that something is not quite right and then you visit us," stressed doctor Pahnke. "But if you had submitted earlier to a related test, the illness would not have developed so badly," concluded doctor Pahnke. In the future, the scientific team at Magdeburg is keen to create a drug (in pill form) from Greek tea: in particular for the variety *sideritis scardica*, which is endemic mainly in Macedonia.

AND IT ACTS AGAINST OSTEOPOROSIS

Laboratory studies on the beneficial effects of mountain tea have already been carried out by the Greek Universities of Patras, and Ioannina; however, a study carried out by the University of Athens (Greece) argues that extracts of *Sideritis euboea* and *Sideritis clandestina* can contribute to prevent osteoporosis, as they protect against the loss of bone density and reinforce the mechanical strength of bone. In the mountains of Greece, there are approximately seventeen native species of mountain tea.

This tea contains a variety of compounds, for example: flavonoids, diterpenes, phenylpropionate, iridoids, and monoterpenes. It also has a stimulating effect and can easily be consumed in the evening before bedtime.

SAGE FOR A HEALTHY BRAIN

Sage (*Salvia officinalis*) is one of the numerous herbs found in Greece. One of the most studied remarkable properties of sage is the effect it can exercise on the functioning of the brain. In a study presented at the British Congress of Pharmacology by King's College of the University of London (UK), it was shown that dried sage roots contain those active ingredients that are similar to those found in modern medications used for the management and treatment of Alzheimer's disease. Indeed, certain ingredients found in sage appeared to inhibit the activity of the enzyme acetylcholinesterase (AChEI), which is found in the brain: this enzyme plays a key role in the development of the disease and in the progressive loss of memory. In addition to the findings of the present study, the findings of a study published in the journal 'Pharmacological Biochemical Behavior' should also be noted: according to this study, it was found that sage has the ability to act as an adjuvant for memory: specifically, the data showed that the extract derived from sage can improve the immediate recall of information.

Let's now have a look in a little more detail at some of the plants and herbs that have been used in Greece for many years for medicinal and culinary purposes.

1. Dittany of Crete (*Origanum dictamnus*)
A Cretan herb known since antiquity; it was used as a haemostatic agent and for healing wounds. Its therapeutic effect on the stomach and its healing properties were mentioned by Hippocrates. Today it mostly consumed as a tisanes.

2. Marjoram (*Origanum microphyllum*)
It has similar properties to thyme, and it has been used since antiquity in treating many cases of nervous disorders; it is also ideal for the treatment of colds.

3. Cretan mountain tea (*Sideritis syriaca*)

It is one of the many types of mountain tea, which are known throughout Greece. In the form of a tisane, it is used as an aid for digestion, as a diuretic, and against colds.

4. Thyme (*Coridothymus capitatus*)
Thyme has antiseptic, diuretic, anti-parasitic, and antipyretic properties: it is also used in cooking to complement various dishes.

5. Winter Savory (*Satureja thymbra*)
The odor resembles that of thyme and oregano. It has both medicinal and apicultural uses. It acts as a sedative in rheumatism, and it is used in cooking.

6. Pink Rock-Rose (*cistus creticus*)
It is an aromatic plant which has medicinal uses. It is effective against insomnia, toothache, and tetanus. Aromatic teas can be made from its leaves.

7. Basil (*Ocimum basilicum*)
It is used as flavouring in foods, and to flavour olive oil either in combination with other herbs or alone. It can relieve migraines, severe headaches, stomatitis, and it soothes abdominal cramps. In the past, it was used in the form of a poultice for soothing stings from scorpions and bees, and nettle rashes.

8. Oregano (*Origanum vulgare*)
This well-known aromatic herb is a fundamental part of the Greek cuisine; it is used with grilled fish, meats, and salads. Its medicinal properties have been known since ancient times. It is used as an appetizer, an antiseptic, and for soothing toothaches and stomach aches. Its essential oil is widely used in perfumery.

9. Chamomile (*Marticaria chamomila*)
This can be used throughout the year. It is usually taken hot as a herbal tea which combines a feeling of perfect relaxation while at the same time combating insomnia. It has several characteristic properties: it can be used as an anti-inflammatory, an anti-allergic, and a palliative agent, and it makes an excellent quality antiseptic.

10. Peppermint (*Mentha x piperita*)

This is considered to be one of the most important herbs. It is used to counter indigestion, nervous disorders, and insomnia. Because of its intense aroma, it is usually used in salads: to which it gives an especially delicious taste. It is usually consumed as a tisane.

11. Small leaved lime (*Tilia cordata Mill*)

This is an aromatic plant that has medicinal properties. The tisane made from its flowers is considered useful in helping digestion. It can also be drunk medicinally as an antitussive, an emollient, an anticonvulsant, a diuretic, a slimming drink, and a diaphoretic.

12. Bay tree (*Laurus nobilis*)

It was formerly used to strengthen the hair, and the tisane was used for the coating those parts of the body that were suffering from rheumatism or muscle contusions. It is very useful for indigestion and for the proper functioning of the stomach. It can also be added to foods for flavouring.

13. Rosemary (*Rosmarinus officinalis*)

As a tisane, it alleviates headaches and is ideal for combating migraines. It is considered by experts that frequent use is ideal for counteracting alopecia. It has antibacterial and antiseptic properties, and it is a very potent stimulant for the circulatory system, as well as a potent potion for insomnia.

14. Common Elder (*Sambucus Nigra*)

The common elder is a valuable herb for combating influenza viruses, colds, and chest ailments.

15. Mint (*Mentha spicata*)

As a tisane it is used as an anticonvulsant, a tonic, and a digestive medication. It is also used to flavour various foods, and toothpaste.

16. Lemon balm (*Melissa officinalis*)

The tisane made with its leaves is considered to have anticonvulsant, anti-inflammatory, and antioxidant properties; additionally, it acts as a heart tonic; it also helps to combat insomnia, and various digestive disorders. It even improves mental clarity.

17. St. John's Wort (*Hypericum perforatum*)
It has several useful properties. It can be used as an anti-inflammatory drug, a styptic drug, a cicatrizing agent, as a sedative, and as an analgesic. It is used in the treatment of neuralgia, and is used as a palliative medicine for sciatic nerve and rheumatic pains. In fact, it is an especially valuable herb in its role either as a cicatrizing agent or as an anti-inflammatory drug.

18. Couch grass (*Agropyron repens*)
As a tisane, it is considered to possess diuretic properties. It has been used in the treatment of cystitis, prostate dysfunction, benign prostatic hypertrophy, nephrolithiasis, and kidney stones. In particular, it is used as a medication for cystitis, and for irritation or inflammation of the ureter.

19. Lemon beebrush (*Lippia citriodora*)
This herb is considered to be highly effective for weight loss while at the same time it combats cellulite. It acts as a palliative medicine for the stomach and the digestive system; it has an antipyretic effect, and the ability to induce a peaceful sleep: free of tension and stress. It is known for its diuretic action, so it is recommended in cases where the body has a tendency to create kidney stones (nephrolithiasis).

20. Pennyroyal (*Mentha pulegium*)
It is a wild plant with a taste reminiscent of mint. It refreshes the palate and helps to revitalize the body. It also helps in digestion and, it is often the favourite 'after dinner' choice.

But it should not be forgotten that sour flavoured foods are equally therapeutic for the body. The eating habits that I had to give up over the years were eating good casserole dishes flavoured with natural lemon juice: whose use in green salads has been replaced by various sweet sauces, as well as artificially prepared lemon juice. I have also read that cinema and pop stars occasionally resort to detox recipes. These recipes must have surely been created by the experts who look after these stars. What, then, is contained in these detox recipes? Lemon and a mixture of herbs! Well, would you believe it? A single forgotten recipe from a plethora of recipes has now become an elixir for the few. Of course, natural lemon juice is especially rich in vitamin C, but it also contains a large number of other vitamins: B1, B2, B3, and B6, proteins, carbohydrates, potassium, and inorganic salts such as calcium, phosphorus, and magnesium. It's not surprising that in olden days it was used to combat scurvy.

It should be noted that potassium is effective in reducing high blood pressure. It is an antipyretic medication, and it is considered one of the most effective natural antimicrobials for combating various viruses, infections, and inflammations.

It should be noted that potassium is effective in reducing high blood pressure. It is an antipyretic medication, and it is considered one of the most effective natural antimicrobials for combating various viruses, infections, and inflammations.

Additionally, lemons (thanks to the abundant content of vitamin C) are ideal for the treatment of winter infections. They are also recommended in diets aimed at controlling cholesterol levels, and for the better wellbeing of the circulatory system.

Drinking lemon juice also helps to alleviate constipation, but its use does not stop there: it helps to maintain the blood vessels in good condition; it is beneficial for our eyesight; it helps the body to absorb iron better; and because it has been demonstrated to function as a diuretic, many people use it when dieting. Finally, it strengthens the gums and is beneficial for the musculoskeletal system: it also helps the musculoskeletal system to absorb calcium better. Lemon juice is a really pleasant 'surprise' for the body, and apart from the necessary flavour that it gives some tasteless foods: it mainly serves to reinforce the body against a number of diseases and infections. How many of you have included lemons and sour flavoured foods in your daily meals?

EAT THE GREEK WAY IF YOU WANT
TO LOSE WEIGHT AND GAIN HEALTH

If you want to be healthy and lose that excess weight forever, the solution for you is the traditional Greek diet, which based on four flavours. The Greek diet is not a recent dietary regimen that has come to prominence because of the results of experimental trials, books, media hype, or endorsements by famous Hollywood stars. Its fame is not due to product marketing; it is a centuries old diet: stretching back to ancient Greek times. This diet includes natural sweet, salty, bitter, and sour flavours: and it protects the body from chronic diseases and promotes longevity.

In ancient Greece, this diet operated mainly as a medicine for the human body: it acted as a healing agent for diseases; whereas, nowadays it is only a means of pleasure and addiction: when you consume food, on the on hand it functions to regenerates the body and on the other hand it functions to limit diseases. (*See ref. 4*)

Indeed, the vehicle for a comprehensive therapeutic diet is flavour. According to Aristotle: "In each case, beneficial food is considered to be sweet flavoured food that is sweet either of itself or as a result of combination with other foods," whereas "salty and bitter-tasting food reduce the severity of disease."

Every historical era has been dominated by two flavours, for example: in Roman times – the bitter and the sweet; in Byzantium times – the sweet and salty; in Ottoman times – the salty and sweet; and in modern times – the sweet and salty. Only in classical Greek antiquity were the four flavors equally prevalent. (*See ref. 5*)

The reader may be interested in knowing about the natural diet of the ancient Greeks, so here is a brief review of their diet.

The staple foods of ancient Greece – with peak from 2000 BC until 300 BC – form what we now call the 'Mediterranean triad': cereals, olive oil, and wine. These staples along with greens, fruits, and vegetables constituted by 70 – 75% of their daily routine. The remaining 25 – 30% was made up of meat and animal by products such as eggs, and goat's milk and cheese.

The main cereal was barley, and various products made from einkorn and emmer wheat, millet, and vetch. From these cereals they made bread, and pies with cheese or honey, and gruel. The bread was eaten with vegetables, and some of the vegetables that have been recorded are wild greens, artichokes, radishes, scallions, garlic, fennel, sweet pea, cabbage, lettuce, chard, nettles, and bulbs.

The pulses that were eaten were lentils, beans, fava, split peas, chickpeas, lupins, and ervil. The fruits were eaten were apples, pears, quinces, cranberries, pomegranates, grapes, plums, blackberries, figs, cranberries, cherries, dates, and lotus plants.

The nuts of that period were almonds, walnuts, sesame seeds, chestnuts, acorns, pine seeds, chestnuts, and flax.

The daily herbs were mint, thyme, oregano, coriander, cumin, capers, rosemary, and cardamom.

Fish was accorded a special place, and since ancient times Greeks have always consumed more fish than that meat. The ancient Greeks ate many varieties of fish: mackerel, sardines, swordfish, tuna, smelt, sea bream, perch, bass, octopus, cuttlefish, squid, lobsters, crayfish, and eels.

Meat was eaten at public and private celebrations. They ate deer, roe deer, wlld boars, hares, partridges, quails and poultry, goats, piglets, and snails.

Finally, like nowadays, the ancient Greeks also snacked: they ate sweet fruits, honey, raisins, and fresh or dried figs.

Many of the above mentioned foods are now classed as superfoods; however, they have been 'abandoned' due to the industrialization and globalization of food processing and cultivation. Until 1970, Greece had fed itself sufficiently on the foods of the ancient Greek and in particular with a diet containing the four flavors; however, now in 2015, the diet of Greek urban dwellers has seen the disappearance of the following foods: snails, fish, eels, millet, gruel, frumenty, barley, most herbs, garlic, onions (due to aesthetics – their smell) cranberries, quinces, figs, cranberries, berries, lotus, sesame, chestnuts, acorns, flax seed, pine nuts, beans, split peas, lupins, ervil, a variety of herbs drinks, raisins, molasses, and must (ancient Greek grape).

Their place – for those who still cook rather than order readymade meals – has been taken over by fatty pre-processed meats, high fat yellow cheeses, white bread, butter, potatoes, tomatoes, corn, peppers, apples, bananas, oranges, mandarins, rice, pasta, mashed potato, and pulses (chickpeas, lentils, and beans): the last item due to the economic crisis. And of course all sorts of coffee, choc-olate drinks, sweets, and snacks with sugar and salt; that is, food with only two flavours – sweet and salty.

Greek cuisine is 'awash' in its most fundamental ingredient – olive oil. It is also a diet which scientists from around the world recommend as a way of life. (*See ref. 6*) The secret of this diet is the 'marriage' of olive oil (which contains unsaturated fats) and vegetables (which contain nitrite (NO_2-) and nitrate (NO_3-) salts): this combination produces a group of nitro fatty acids which helps to lower blood pressure. (*See ref. 7*)

Also, olive oil and fiber reduce appetite and create a sensation of satiation in the brain. A few drops of unrefined olive oil added to salads or food increase the sensation of satiation which assists in lowering calorie intake by 200 calories. (*See ref. 8*)

But fiber, which is found in fruits, vegetables, and whole grains, also plays an important role: it retards the accumulation of excess weight. (*See ref. 9*)

The study of this diet has produced some unique medical findings: the first time in Crete in 1960, then five years ago in Ikaria – even though this has been the dietary system of the monastic community of Mount Athos for hundreds of years.

All three regions eat foods of the same flavours: olive oil (bitter), fruits (sour, sweet, and bitter), herbs (bitter), vegetables (sweet and bitter), legumes (sweet), whole meal bread (salty and bitter), fish (sweet), a few dairy products (sweet and sour), eggs (sweet), a minimal amount of red meat (sweet), herbs (bitter) and Greek tisanes (bitter).

The inhabitants of all three regions observe periods of fasting: in combination, these periods amount to an annual total of 170 days. During these periods of fasting, they abstain from meat, fish, milk, cheese, eggs, olive oil, and desserts or sweets made with butter or eggs. Fasting is, effectively, a detoxifying process that is engaged in for almost half of each year on an annual basis.

The Greek balanced diet along with exercise and abstinence from smoking not only reduces the risk of premature death: it also increases life expectancy for women by fifteen years and that for men by eight years. (*See ref. 10*)

The medical community has conducted a lot of research on the Greek diet and its beneficial effects on human health. Let's now look at three cases that have dominated the news worldwide.

1 THE IKARIAN SECRET CODE OF LIFE

In guidebooks, Ikaria is depicted as an island with beautiful beaches, wonderful local produce, and representative of a typical picturesque Greek holiday location. Indeed, for tourists, Ikaria is a place that has its own pace – they call it the 'Jamaica' of the Aegean. It is an island whose inhabitants don't follow the conventional Greek norms, for example: while in other regions of Greece the pace is fast and stressful, everything here is so laid-back. And whereas elsewhere family relationships are on the wane, in Ikaria families and friends support anyone who has a problem.

The island of Ikaria is of particular interest for doctors because whereas in the rest of Europe only 0.1% of the population lives beyond ninety years of age, in Ikaria the figure is tenfold (National Statistical Services of Greece).

Over six years ago, scientific data showed that Ikaria (Greece), Sardinia, Loma Linda (USA), Nicoya (Costa Rica), and Okinawa (Japan) were the regions with the highest percentage of old people.

To date, the observations of the medical research group in Ikaria (*See ref. 11*) have arrived at the conclusion that, apart from the diet, the lifestyle of the inhabitants acts in a protective capacity against the incidence of cardiovascular and neo-plastic diseases: it seems that the long-term consumption of raw foodstuffs in conjunction with siestas and the control of stress are contributory factors.

So, what are they doing in Ikaria? In terms of diet, they eat fruits, vegetables, fish, legumes, meat (although rarely), and on a daily basis they drink olive oil, mountain tea, and one or two cups of Greek coffee.
A typical day would include the following:

For breakfast: goat's milk, mountain tea or coffee, honey, and bread.

For lunch: almost always beans (lentils, chickpeas), potatoes, vegetables (fennel, dandelion, green vegetables), and any seasonal garden vegetables.

For dinner: bread and goat's milk.

And if you are curious about Christmas and Easter: they slaughter the family pigs and thereby enjoy small servings of cured pork for several months throughout the year. (*See ref. 12*)

Whatever else they may or may not do – they drink mountain tea daily. This is made from dried herbs that grow on the island, and the drink is enjoyed by the inhabitants of Ikaria as "a cocktail to end the day." They even drink wild marjoram, sage, pennyroyal, rosemary, and a drink made by boiling dandelions to which a little lemon is then added. (*See ref.13*) *These teas are also traditional Greek remedies for various ailments, and they have been used by successive generations of Ikarians.*

At the same time, the researchers have also uncovered another secret of longevity; this lies in the way the inhabitants of Ikaria prepare Greek coffee. According to the experts, the slow boiling of coffee on hot ash results in a final product that contains more antioxidants (polyphenols) than coffee that is brought to the boil quickly: the important point of all this being that polyphenols are beneficial for the cardiovascular system.

But the good health of the inhabitants of Ikaria also derives from what they don't eat. For example, white flour and sugar are either consumed in very small amounts or not at all, and processed sweet and savoury flavoured foods are not included in the diet. To reiterate, their diet is based on four flavours that are found in foodstuffs such as olive oil, olives, herbs, vegetables, coffee (bitter), fruit (sweet and sour), fish, and little red meat (sweet). This 'cocktail' of flavours promotes longevity, reduced stress, makes one more optimistic, gives one a feeling of purpose in life, and helps in the detoxification of the body during periods of fasting. The 'miracle' of longevity in Ikaria has been the subject of many detail reports by media outlets such as 'The BBC', 'The New York Times', 'The Financial Times', 'The Guardian', 'The Australian', 'ABC News', 'The Daily Mail', and 'NBC News' to mention but a few.

2 THE AGE-OLD CRETANS

Crete, the island of Zeus, is a beautiful Greek island situated on the edge of the eastern Aegean Sea; it is an island that God has bestowed with all things good. In 1960, a study was conducted by the American scientist Ancel Keys in Crete and six other world locations on the role played by lifestyles and diets on cardiovascular diseases.

In the survey, Keys compared the diets of 12,763 male inhabitants from Greece (the islands of Crete and Corfu), Yugoslavia, Italy, Netherlands, Finland, USA, and Japan. The results showed that the inhabitants of Crete had the highest longevity in the world.

When, thirty-one years after the start of the study, the Department of Public Health of the University of Crete conducted medical examinations on the Cretan participants: approximately 50% were still alive; however, there was not even one living participant from the other six countries (inclusive of the participants from the rest of Greece). Scientists believe that the cause of this extraordinary health is due to the Cretan diet.

What, then, is the diet that is the key to the secret of Cretan longevity? It is the diet which contains a lot of olive oil, vegetables, and fruits: and to a lesser extent, cheese, milk, eggs, seafood, snails, a little white meat, red meat (very rarely), and a little red wine with every meal. To these foods, one can also add legumes (such as beans, lentils, and split peas), and bread (containing a minimum of two types of flour: wheat and oats). Of course, they did not use sugar – fruit and honey were preferred. Moreover, they also used local herbs in cooking and in making herbal teas. In fact, they ate foods that contained the four flavours: mostly bitter flavoured foods, and in the case of sweet flavoured foods – only in their natural forms.

A typical daily diet would be as follows:

For breakfast: mountain tea with honey, homemade bread, and homemade cheese.

For brunch: bread with olives and grapes.

For lunch: snails with cracked wheat, salad (tomato, cucumber, or carrot), bread, a glass of red wine, and two apples.

For dinner: chips fried in olive oil, wild greens, bread, a glass of red wine, and an apple.

A typical Sunday diet would be as follows:
For breakfast: Greek coffee, cheese pies with honey, and 2 oranges.
For lunch: lamb or goat with tomato and potatoes, salad (tomato, cucumber, or carrot) bread, a glass of red wine, and an apple.

For dinner: omellete (with potatoes, tomatoes, or peppers), salad (tomato, lettuce, or carrot), bread, a glass of red wine, and a pear. (*See ref. 14*)

Another study, the Lyon Diet Heart Study, was more revealing in its findings concerning the Cretan diet. The study involved 600 people who had suffered a first myocardial infarction. Half were given the Cretan diet enriched with omega-3 fatty acids, and the other half the diet recommended by the American Heart Association.

The study had originally been set to run for 48 months; however, it was terminated after 27 months, because the difference between the two groups was so great that it was deemed unethical to continue.

The 300 participants who were on the Cretan diet had 76% fewer heart attacks (second episode) compared with the group that was on the diet prescribed by the American Heart Association. These results were so impressive that to date they have not been achieved either by the use of invasive surgery or by pharmaceutical methods. (See ref. 15)

Another characteristic feature here, as in Ikaria, is the role played by fasting in the daily life of the Cretans: they also fast annually for about 170 days in total.
Articles and reports about the Cretan diet have been published in the many magazines, scientific journals, and reported by the mass media. Of particular interest is the experience of photojournalist Matthieu Paley of the National Geographic who has described the preparation of a Cretan menu: he accompanied an eighty year old woman who picked wild greens (many with bitter tastes) for the purpose of making 'kalitsounia': pies made with wild greens. When he later sat down to eat the snails, sardines, beans, barley, and rusks that had been laid out on the table, a Cretan showed him a small plate and said, "This is a medicine. Medicine! Eat a lot of it!"
I try to get a sense of the flavour described by Matthieu Paley. It's a little bitter, the kind of bitter that I sense is good for you. (See ref. 16)

3 THE MIRACLE OF MOUNT ATHOS
Mount Athos, which has been in existence for over a millennium, is a small autonomous region of the Greek State located on the easternmost part of the Khalkidhiki peninsula: it consists of twenty principal monasteries, and twelve hermitages that make up the Holy Community. The monastic community can

be visited, but only by males, and permission must be obtained prior to visiting: access to women is absolutely forbidden. Life there has barely changed since AD 963, and a monk's life there could best be described as a Spartan existence: but it is this way of life in which is the hidden secret of the monks' longevity. Medical monitoring of the monks has revealed a very low incidence of cancer, heart diseases, and Alzheimer's disease. Furthermore, they were found live up to ninety-five years of age while still retaining good mental and physical health. What is their daily prescription for longevity, then?

- The alternation of days of fasting with non-fasting days: for at least half the days of the year, the monks abstain from eating certain foods and olive oil.
- In general, they do not eat meat, fat, or spices.
- Their diet includes olive oil, fish, legumes, vegetables, fruits, olives, whole grain bread, Tahini (sesame paste), halva, tea, wild greens, berry plants (such as wild strawberries, blueberries, and cranberries), and chestnuts.
- The establishment of a dietary regimen based on two daily meals instead of three as in the Western world: the monks only eat once in the morning and once in the evening unlike westerners who have breakfast, lunch, tea, and, dinner.
- Daily, they engage in manual work required for the upkeep of the monasteries.
- They consume the local herbs.

"The miracle of life on Mount Athos" was also the subject of CBS News's '60 minutes' programme. After on the spot reporting, the presenter commented that since they (the monks) didn't have many diseases, they were probably doing something right.

The diet of the monks of Mount Athos was also dealt with in an article which was published in a supplement of the Danish newspaper 'Berlingske Tidende' under the title of "Eat like a monk and avoid cancer".
According to Stig Ekkert – the Danish doctor who had visited the monks of Mount Athos – these monks rarely exhibited cancer. The article was published on the front page of the supplement (titled: "The monk's anti-cancer diet", and subtitled: "The monks of the Greek peninsula of Mount Athos are free from can-

cer") with a full-page photo of a monk from Mount Athos, who is shown holding a lobster and a crayfish in his hands. Interestingly, this region is often visited by Vladimir Putin and Prince Charles and many other famous men and, as the newspapers covering the story say: "they must know something more."

So once again, we have here the same recipe for longevity: the diet of four flavours.

But the 'beauty' of the flavours in the monks' diet does not derive from the variety of foods, or the spices, or even elaborate ways of cooking. The flavors are authentic, and they include all four flavours: bitter (e.g. tahini, herbs, olive oil, olives, greens, wild fruits), salty (e.g. bread), sweet (e.g. legumes, fish, and fruit), and sour (e.g. lemons (fruit), or sourdough bread).

References

1. Lionis C. et al. (1998). Antioxidant effects of herbs in Crete. The Lancet 1998; 352.

2. Mendel V. Ex situ preservation and marketing of Greek endemic plants. (Mendel is a silvicul-turalist by profession.)

3. Geromichalou George D. (Currently he is head of the Cell Culture Molecular Modeling & Drug Design Lab, Symeonidion Research Centre, Theagenion Cancer Hospital, Greece).

4. Aristotle's "On sensing and feeling", Chapter 4, 442a.

5. George Boskos professor at the University of Athens Harokopion Nutrition & Dietetics.

6. Huffington Post article.

7. Research by the University of California (USA), and King's College, University of London (UK).

8. Research by the Technical University of Munich (Germany), and the University of Vienna (Austria).

9. Tests on mice by researchers from the Imperial College, University of London (UK).

10. Study by the University of Maastricht (Holland).

11. The team was led by Christodoulos Stefanadis, professor of cardiology at the University of Athens and Director of the First Cardiology Clinic at the Hippocratic University Hospital. Research: June – October, 2009 – 2010.

12. New York Times article.

13. Doctor Elias Iliadis's statement to the New York Times.

14. Kafatos A. Nutrition for the promotion of health and the prevention of chronic diseases (Kafatos is the Professor of Preventive Medicine and Nutrition at the University of Crete, Greece).

15. See 14.

16. http://paleyphoto.photoshelter.com/gallery/Mediterranean-The-Cretans/G00007.wXWP-gnmyU/ and http://www.nationalgeographic.com/foodfeatures/evolution-of-diet/

CHAPTER 4
THE FOUR FLAVOURS DIET

THE PROGRAMME

Before I started the on 'the diet of four flavours', I was in such a state of mind that if I were sat at a table and in front of me there was a nice sweet and salty flavoured cheeseburger and French fries – I would devour it without further thought. I ate because I was stimulated by the sensation of sweet and salty flavours 'exploding' in my mouth. I felt pure pleasure with every mouthful of sauce and fatty food. These rich, full flavours caressed my palate, but after meals I felt such heaviness in my stomach that I just wanted to lie down; and as a result, I was just lolling around all day when I wasn't working.

Today I am going to eat a dish with four flavours, and I shall feel as light as a feather. I shall feel strong, and I shall be able to continue with my day. I am also fully aware that this is the correct 'fuel' for my body. You can think of it like petrol. Do you put petrol in your car that has the correct research octane number (RON) so as to provide more energy and less wear, or do you put whatever petrol you find in front of you?

Since I started on a diet that contains the four flavours, I feel mentally and physically balanced and don't have obsessions. I do not care about how many kilos I will lose; I am interested in gaining my health. And that's because I do not feel deprived of any flavours since at meal times, before my body asks for a particular flavour – I have already provided it. I no longer feel that I have reached the end of my tether or am subject to psychological ups and downs. I am no longer fixated on what I'm going to eat since I now consider each meal like a game: every day, I place the different flavoured foods on my plate next to each other as if doing a jigsaw puzzle.

From the research I had done and the people I had met who were on a traditional Greek diet of four flavours, I realized that they were nourishing themselves as if they were in the phase that experts call the maintenance phase.

HOW I STARTED TO LOSE WEIGHT

Since my teens, I remember that I used to eat in the morning, at noon, and at night: as well as snack regularly between meals. A successful way to initially retard this downward spiral that leads to obesity is to do what I did: write down what you eat. By continuously monitoring what you eat, you will be able to highlight any problems. And these will be solved, if – and I repeat this from personal experience – you record daily the flavours of the foods that you have had. Thus, for instance, you'll know if you are eating only sweet flavoured foods. This way you can adjust your diet accordingly.

In the morning, I, for instance, used to have either two slices of cake (a sweet flavour) because I was anxious to get to work; or I didn't eat eating anything, and I only drank coffee with sugar (a sweet flavour) because I had slept badly; or I neither ate nor drank coffee at home because I was anxious to get to the office.

If you always write down next to each food its flavour, I'm confident you'll get a surprise: you will find, contrary to what you might believe, that sweet and salty flavours predominate.

So, as soon as you realize what you are eating for you breakfast, you can start to make changes so that you get a breakfast that is correctly balanced for flavour. For example, for years I had the following breakfast:

Cake and croissants – SWEET FLAVOUR
Coffee and sugar – SWEET FLAVOUR
Milk with cereals – SWEET FLAVOUR
Nowadays, I have retained only one flavour – the sweet flavour for each day, and I supplement it with the other flavours, viz:

A spoonful of honey – SWEET FLAVOUR
Greek yoghurt – SOUR FLAVOUR
A slice of whole meal bread – SALTY FLAVOUR
Two teaspoons of olive oil – BITTER FLAVOUR

And all of this on a 25 cm diameter plate. It is understood that when I can't have all four flavours in the morning, I keep one or two flavours, accordingly, for lunch at noon or 1 pm. In this way, I don't get hunger pangs or cravings.

So, for instance, I can have fruit (sweet) with yoghurt (sour) and tahini (bitter) and leave the salty flavour for later: this could be a rusk or a slice of whole meal bread. For lunch, one or two flavours on a small 20 cm diameter plate, and the other two or three flavours in a salad bowl, e.g. chicken (sweet) on a small plate, and rocket (bitter) with Greek rusks (salty) and lemon (sour) in a salad bowl; or spaghetti (sweet) on a small plate, and rocket (bitter) with Greek feta (salt) and lemon (sour) in a salad bowl.

Thus, my menu in accordance with the Greek diet is as follows:

White meat once a week
Spaghetti or rice once a week
Fish twice a week
Legumes three times a week

These have naturally sweet flavours and are eaten on a small (20 cm diameter) plate. They are always accompanied by a rich salad made up of foods that contain the other three flavours; this is eaten from a salad bowl.

Throughout the day, I have the following:

Three servings of sweet flavoured food (e.g. meat, fish, pulses, pasta foods, rice, eggs) or fruit (e.g. apples, bananas, pears, grapes, water melon).

Three servings of salty flavoured food whose portions are the size of a mobile phone (not a mobile tablet): e.g. cheese, bread, and rusks.

Three servings of sour flavoured food (e.g. fruit, bread or rusks made with sour-dough, Greek yoghurt, or lemon juice) and

Three servings of bitter flavoured food (salads, olive oil, olives, or wild fruits).

I also drink lots of Greek drinks and, at the most, two Greek coffees in a small espresso sized cup without sugar: all the drinks are bitter flavoured.

And for dinner, I repeat my breakfast on a 25 cm diameter plate, or if I am really hungry, I repeat my lunch.

My diet became simple, natural, with variety, and measured in quantity. In other words, what I eat has not been affected by the food processing industry; therefore, it has retained its nutrients.

The 'game' with the four flavours will give you the solution to enable you to fix your diet. First choose what foods you like to eat and put them in one of the four flavours categories: sweet, salty, bitter, or sour. At the end of the book, you will find a list of foods which, along with any others you may like to eat, should also be placed in one of the four flavours categories. In this way, you will have a diet plan ready with the foods that you like. Finding the category that a particular food falls into is easy because your guide is – flavour.

STAGE 1 (15 DAYS)

FOOD DIARY – I ONLY ATE WHEN I WAS HUNGRY

From my experience, this stage is the most important. If you succeed in this part, you will lose weight without realizing it. Your brain will try to make you do various things, for example: in the past, it used to instruct me to "Stuff it!", "Gobble it up!", "Eat more!", and other similar instructions. Nowadays, however, my brain acts as a brake: "You're not going to eat again, are you?", "And what do you intend to eat?", "You can always eat later." and so on. You have to understand that the diary of flavours is the mirror of your diet: in it you can see what you are eating and what you are doing wrong on a daily basis. If your brain records it, it will change your whole life.

To reiterate: you must conscientiously follow your diary of flavours. Record the flavour and if you wish, how you felt, i.e. the feeling that was aroused in you. In this way you may be able to determine which feelings are associated with each flavour. In the beginning you will view it with surprise (as I did); then, you will get annoyed: but in the end, you will be positively surprised by both the quantities you will consume and the flavours you will taste.

After having completed the process of recording your bad habits, you will have to realize that you must eat only when you are hungry. And you should always be on the lookout for any other bad habits, which you should correct, for example: I noticed that I ate excessively when I was with friends; I felt relaxed; I was comfortable in their company, so I didn't stop to think about how much food I was eating. Another bad habit of mine was that I ate a lot of snacks when I was at work: due to the stress of having to visit various companies during my working day, I found myself eating biscuits, sweets, pastries, buns, chocolates, and other sweet foods. I would eat a selection of everything, but towards the end of the day I was still left feeling hungry – so I would eat again, but then I would end up feeling bloated.

I had a similar problem when I was at home. I felt relaxed, so I would decide not to have a meal. I would pour myself a drink and just eat a few assorted nuts; half an hour later, I would pour myself another drink and eat a few more assorted nuts. But then, I had hunger pangs, so I just ate whatever I found that could be prepared quickly, or I order a meal from a takeaway. In the end, I just changed these habits with new ones: the good thing is that new habits form new routines – and these replace your previous bad habits. For example, now when I'm with friends, I fill up my plate with foods that contain the four flavours, but I don't eat anything else. At work, I have ceased snacking: I only eat fruit or a large Greek rusk. And if you'd like to know – I now feel better, sleep better, and wake up incredibly full of energy.

Also, my diary of flavours blocks the excessive consumption of starch and retards the over consumption of protein. In fact, it regulates the consumption of all the categories of foodstuffs.

Summary & Goals

In the morning, I had whatever I liked served on a 25 cm diameter plate. For lunch, I had whatever I liked but served on a 20 cm diameter plate and a salad served in a salad bowl. For dinner, again I had whatever I liked served on a 25 cm diameter plate. The aim of this stage is to see what flavours you are consuming and to learn how to use the different sized plates which act as a measure of the amount of food that you consume.

Here's a simple layout for your food diary: repeat the layout for each day of the week.

MONDAY

FOOD EATEN – TASTE – REASON FOR EATING IT (HABIT)

Morning

Lunch

Dinner

STAGE 2 (1 MONTH)

DETYOXIFICATION – I WEANED MYSELF OFF SALT & SUGAR

Before you can make a new start, you'll have to ditch your bad habits. So, you'll have to wean yourself off refined sugar and salty flavours – and it's not an easy thing to do; it took me a whole month. During that period it was as if I were on a see-saw: one minute I would be off the bad old diet and on the good new diet, and then the next minute I would be back on the bad old diet and off the good new diet, and so on. What got me weaned off refined sugar was replacing it with natural sweet flavours: so, whenever I craved for something sweet, I would have an apple, or a pear, a mature lotus, or a banana, or some Greek yoghurt with half a teaspoonful of honey. I had also stopped putting refined sugar in my coffee: in the first week, it tasted like poison; I couldn't drink it, but in the end – I got used to it. And instead of fizzy drinks, I only drank tisanes made with Greek herbs – which I drank without any sugar.

The foods I removed and the foods I replaced them with:

- Fizzy drink were replaced by tisanes without sugar
- Chocolates were replaced by doughnuts
- Sweet cakes were replaced by ice-cream
- Sugary sweets and cakes were replaced by sweet fruits, tahini with honey, or Greek yoghurt with honey or dry fruits or raisins.
- Coffee with refined white sugar was replaced by coffee without sugar

Weaning myself off salty flavours was easier for me. I had become so used to adding a lot of white salt in order to get a strong flavour that anyone looking at my food would have thought it had been left out in the snow. So, the first thing I did was to substitute herbs for salt. Thus, instead of being a heavily salted food, it became intensely aromatic. These herbal products are, by composition, 20% crude salt mixed with an 80% herbal combination of thyme, savory, garlic, pepper, basil, oregano, rosemary, mint, marjoram, spearmint, linseed, and sesame. The salt used is unprocessed and is naturally found in sea water or in mineral form. The salt and herbs mixture is a natural product which also contains trace elements and minerals.

You too can easily make your own salt and herbs seasoning. Choose the herbs you like, buy them in dried form (not fresh), and grind them all together using a mortar and pestle, or a grinding mill. After you have ground all the herbs together, add the crude salt and grind the mixture again. Finally, put the ground mixture in a salt shaker – it is now ready for use. (In the RECIPES section, I have recommended the Mediterranean flavoured seasonings which I make.)

Later, I completely removed salt from my food and added more herbs. So now, I have all my foods with plain herbs. Besides, salt can be indirectly obtained from many other foods: from bread, cheese, and other foods that should be, with moderation, included in your diet.

The foods I removed and the foods I replaced them with:

- Savoury snacks were replaced by unsalted nuts
- Refined salt was replaced by a mixture of herbs and unrefined salt
- Salt with herbs was replaced by plain herbs

Summary & Goals

I substituted a mixture of crude salt and herbs for refined salt. Later I substituted plain herbs for crude salt and herbs. I substituted Greek herbs and green tea for fizzy drinks, and I substituted fruit, honey, and raisins for sugar. For breakfast, I had whatever I liked served on a 25 cm diameter plate. For lunch, I had whatever I liked, but served on a 20 cm diameter plate, and a salad in a salad bowl. For dinner, again I had whatever I liked served on a 25 cm diameter plate. The aim of this stage is to stop the consumption of refined sugar and salt and to replace them with natural sugars, and unrefined salt and herbs, respectively.

STAGE 3 (15 DAYS)

CHANGES TO BREAKFAST & DINNER

I have always had breakfast and dinner on a 25 cm diameter plate. At this stage, I started to have meals that contained all the four flavours, for example: sour flavours were provided by fruit and yoghurt; salty flavours from bread and cheese; bitter flavours from tahini with olive oil; and sweet flavours from honey or dried fruits. (For more options see the list below or create your own list.) I worked for fifteen days on the breakfast and the dinner in order to create a large variety of choices. Breakfast and dinner can be the same if you're tired and not very hungry. Sometimes when I was very hungry, I used to have the same food for dinner as I had had for lunch.

BREAKFAST – The foods I removed and the foods I replaced them with:

Patisserie sweets were replaced by fruit (sweet)
Cornflakes was replaced by tahini (bitter)
Rusks (salty or sour)
Marmalades
Cakes made with olive oil (bitter)
Beverages (bitter)
Bacon, lemon (sour)
Yoghurt (sour)
Pancakes
Sausages, honey (sweet)
Potatoes
Biscuits

DINNER – The foods I removed and the foods I replaced them with:

Variety pizza was replaced by fruit (sour/sweet)
Ready-made food was replaced by salad (bitter)
Crisps were replaced by yoghurt (sour)
Alternatively, you can have the lunchtime food again.

Summary & Goals

I replaced the two flavours with healthy choices of sweet and salty flavoured foods, and added the other two flavours: bitter and sour. I had breakfast on a 25 cm diameter plate, and I also used the same sized plate for dinner for a meal consisting of food containing all four flavours: but if I was really hungry, I would have the same food for dinner as I had had for lunch. The aim of this step is to integrate all 4 flavours – but ONLY in the breakfast and dinner.

STAGE 4 (15 DAYS)

CHANGES TO LUNCH

And now we come to lunch. The problem is if, like me, you work intensively and get used to having lunch after work: will you have the strength and patience to prepare it? Perhaps, you'll even have to re-plan your daily diet schedule. I would insist on re-planning because once you find the foods that belong to one of the four categories – you can start the 'game' of four flavors.

I always have lunch on a 20 cm diameter plate when I have meat, fish, legumes, rice, or spaghetti, and the salad is eaten from a salad bowl. In traditional Greek cuisine, there are foods in which the four flavours can be mixed together. These foods are part of the diet of the three areas I have already mentioned: Crete, Ikaria, and (to a lesser extent) Mount Athos.

LUNCH – The foods I removed and the foods I replaced them with:

Red meat was replaced by white meat – once a week
Salad was replaced by greens (bitter)
Fatty cheese was replaced by legumes (sweet)
Fatty foods were replaced by oily foods (sweet, sour)
Fish (sweet)
Chips were replaced by olive oil (bitter)
Pickles were replaced by herbs (bitter)
Soft drinks were replaced by rice (sweet)
Butter was replaced by boiled or roast potatoes (sweet)
White bread was replaced by whole meal bread (sour, salty)
Syrups and sauces were replaced by lemons with olive oil and herbs (sour or bitter)

Summary & Goals

For lunch, the food that contained two flavours was eaten on a 20 cm diameter plate, and the food that contained the other two or three flavours was eaten from a salad bowl. The aim is to have a lunch that contains all four flavours.

AND FOR THE LADIES?

The attitude of women towards someone who is slimming is of some interest. Some of my female friends who noticed that I had lost weight asked me outright in front of others how I had managed it; whereas, other female friends asked me in private. When I started to explain the thinking behind the diet programme, they liked it; they found it logical and playful, and some of them asked for the diet programme: they wanted me to give them the list of foods that I had drawn up for breakfast, lunch, and dinner. After a while, whenever we met, they never brought up the subject again; but this attitude changed as soon as the diet had produced visible results; then, they fully revealed the recipe for their success: they followed what I had done, but for breakfast and dinner, they had used a smaller plate – a fruit plate, which is 20cm in diameter.

That ate meals containing all four flavours for breakfast and dinner on a 20 cm diameter plate, and at lunchtime a meal containing one or two flavours again on a 20 cm diameter plate and the other two or three flavours from food in a salad bowl. However, overall, they consumed less than I did.

Maria, Dionysia, Sarah, Vassia, Demeter, Katherine, Christina, Niki, and Vaso are some of my female friends who lost weight and now feel much better because of it.

THE PROGRAMME
FOR MEN & WOMEN

STAGE 1 (15 DAYS)

KEEP A FOOD DIARY & LEARN ABOUT WHAT YOU EAT & ONLY EAT WHEN YOU ARE HUNGRY

Note: It took me 15 days. In the reader's case, it may be more or less.

At this stage you should keep a food diary of the different foods (and their flavours) that you eat, and your daily dietary habits. The goal is to determine why you eat sweet and salty flavoured foods and your psychological condition when you consume these foods. Once you realize what your problem is, you will eat only when you are hungry: irrespective of whether it is morning, afternoon, or evening.

MEN
For breakfast, you can have whatever you want served on a 25 cm diameter plate. For lunch, you can also have whatever you want, but served on a 20 cm diameter plate along with a salad served in a salad bowl. Finally, for dinner, again you can have whatever you want served on a 25 cm diameter plate. The aim of this stage is to see what flavours you are consuming and to learn how to use the different sized plates which act as a measure of the amount of food that you consume.

WOMEN
Irrespective of whether it is breakfast, lunch or dinner, you can eat whatever you want on a 20 cm diameter plate: lunch should also include a salad served in a salad bowl.

STAGE 2 (1 MONTH)

WEANING YOURSELF OFF SALT & SUGAR

What to eat and what not to eat:

Instead of Soft drinks drink plain tisanes.
Instead of Chocolates, donuts, patisserie sweets, ice creams, sweets, and cakes eat sweet fruits, yoghurt (with honey or dry fruits, or raisins), or tahini with honey.
Instead of coffee with refined white sugar drink bitter coffee.
Instead of salty snacks eat salt free nuts.
Instead of refined salt use herbs.
Instead of raw salt and herbs use a mixture of pure herbs.

Substitute a mixture of raw salt and herbs for refined salt: later, you can use a mixture of various herbs without any salt. Substitute Greek herbs and green tea for soft drinks, and substitute fruit, honey, raisins and naturally occurring sweet flavoured foods for refined white sugar: this way, you will eliminate refined white sugar from your diet.
The goal of this stage is to stop the consumption of refined sugar and salt and to replace them accordingly with natural sugars, and unrefined salt and herbs.

MEN

For breakfast, you can have whatever you want served on a 25 cm diameter plate. For lunch, you can also have whatever you want, but served on a 20 cm diameter plate along with a salad served in a salad bowl. Finally, for dinner, again you can have whatever you want served on a 25 cm diameter plate

WOMEN

Irrespective of whether it is breakfast, lunch or dinner, you can eat whatever you want on a 20 cm diameter plate: lunch should also include a salad served in a salad bowl.

STAGE 3 (15 DAYS)

THE FOUR FLAVOURS FOR BREAKFAST & DINNER

The aim of this step is to integrate all four flavours – but ONLY in the breakfast and dinner.

MEN

Foods containing all four flavours are eaten for breakfast and dinner on a 25 cm diameter plate. For lunch, eat whatever you want, but served on a 20 cm diameter plate along with a salad served in a salad bowl.

WOMEN

Foods containing all four flavours are eaten for breakfast and dinner on a 20 cm diameter plate. For lunch, eat whatever you want, again served on a 20 cm diameter plate along with a salad served in a salad bowl.

STAGE 4 (15 DAYS)

THE FOUR FLAVOURS FOR LUNCH

MEN

For lunch, the food that contains two flavours is eaten on a 20 cm diameter plate, and the food that contains the other two or three flavours is eaten from a salad bowl. The aim is to have a healthy lunch that contains all four flavours.

WOMEN

For lunch, the food that contains two flavours is eaten on a 20 cm diameter plate, and the food that contains the other two or three flavours is eaten from a salad bowl. The aim is to have a healthy lunch that contains all four flavours.

If you feel ready, you can go directly to stage 3 and 4 and at the same time apply stage 1 and 2. That is, if you decide to start by changing your breakfast and dinner, you must also simultaneously cease using salt and sugar.
You can then keep your food diary for as long as you wish.

QUICK GREEK DIET RECIPES FOR BREAKFAST & DINNER

(These twenty recipes are served on a 25 cm diameter plate for men
and a 20 cm diameter plate for women)

[KEY ds: dessert spoon; ss: soup spoon.]

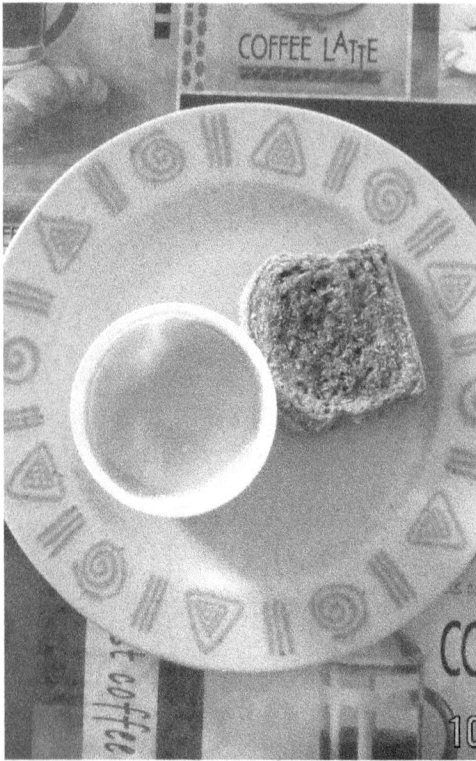

RECIPE 1

SWEET
1 ds of Honey

SOUR
1 Greek yoghurt

SALTY
1 rusk

BITTER
1 ss of olive oil with oregano

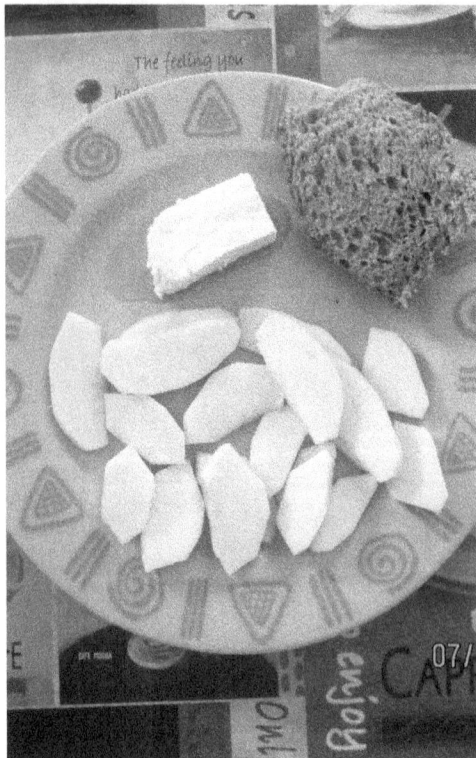

RECIPE 2

SWEET
1 apple

SOUR
1 slice of bread

SALTY
1 piece of feta cheese

BITTER
1 ss of olive oil with oregano

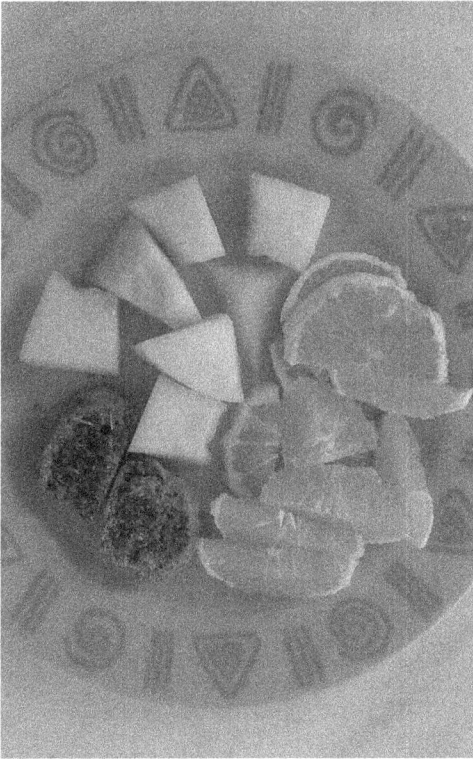

RECIPE 3

SWEET
2-3 pieces of melon

SOUR
1 orange

SALTY
1 rusk

BITTER
1 ss of olive oil with oregano

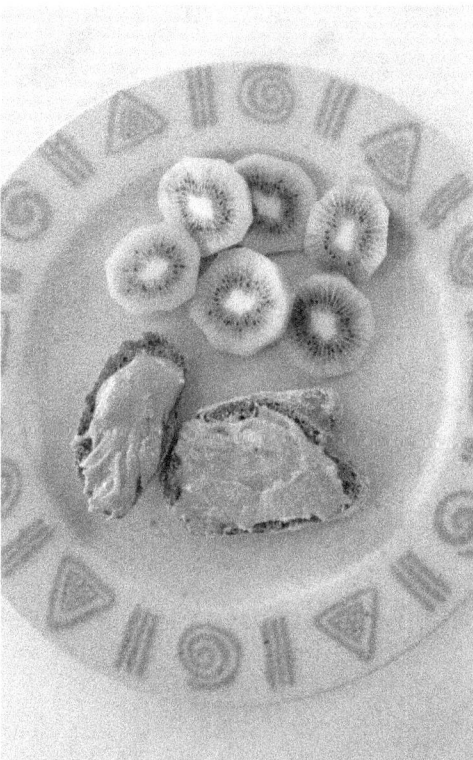

RECIPE 4

SWEET
1 ss of honey

SOUR
1 Kiwi

SALTY
1 slice of bread

BITTER
1 ss of Tahini

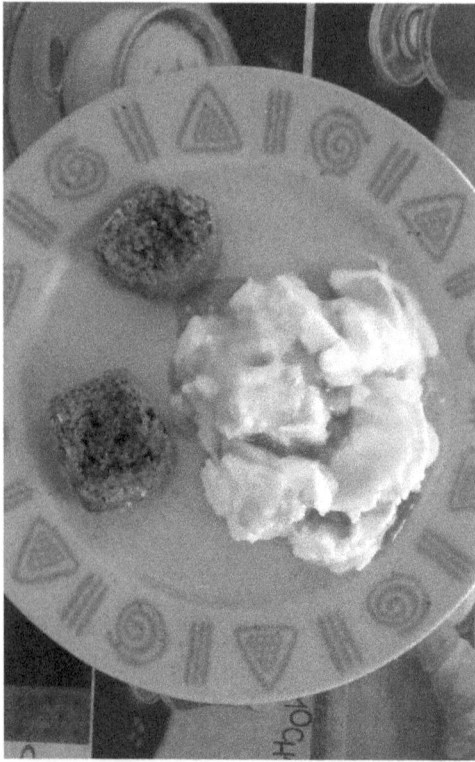

RECIPE 5

SWEET
1 ss of honey

SOUR
1 Greek yoghurt

SALTY
1 rusk

BITTER
1 ss of olive oil with oregano

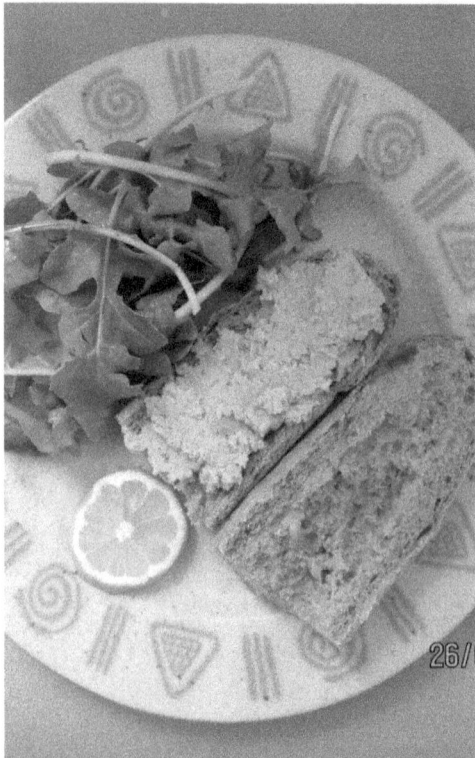

RECIPE 6

SWEET
Fava bean paste

SOUR
A few drops of lemon

SALTY
1 slice of bread

BITTER
Rocket and olive oil

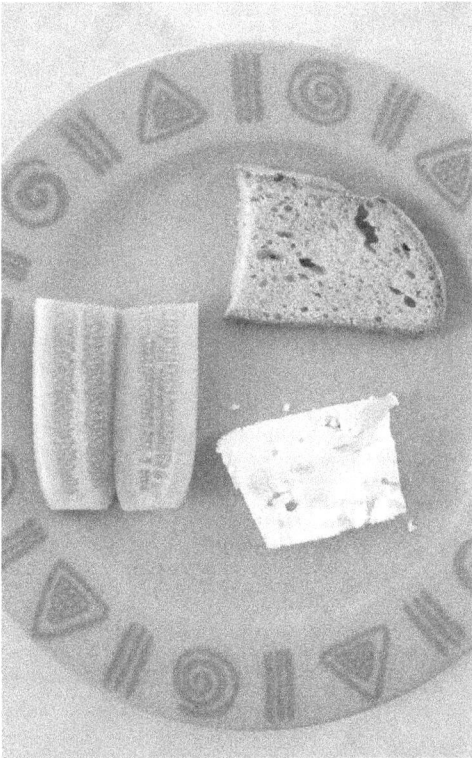

RECIPE 7

SWEET
1 cucumber

SOUR
1 slice of bread

SALTY
1 piece of feta cheese

BITTER
1 ss of olive oil with oregano

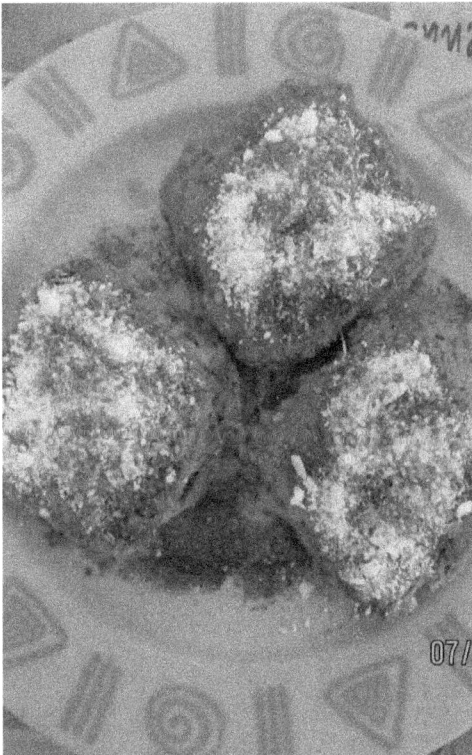

RECIPE 8

SWEET
1 piece of cream cheese

SOUR
Half a tomato

SALTY
1 rusk

BITTER
1 ss of olive oil with oregano

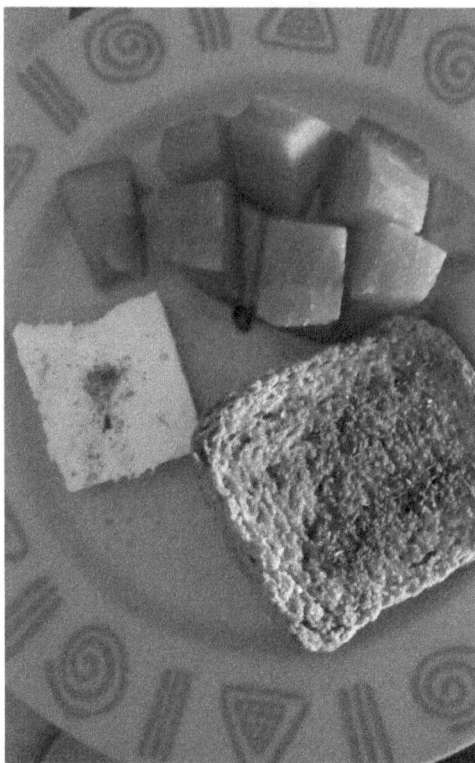

RECIPE 9

SWEET
2 pieces of watermelon

SOUR
1 rusk

SALTY
1 piece of feta cheese

BITTER
1 ss of olive oil with oregano

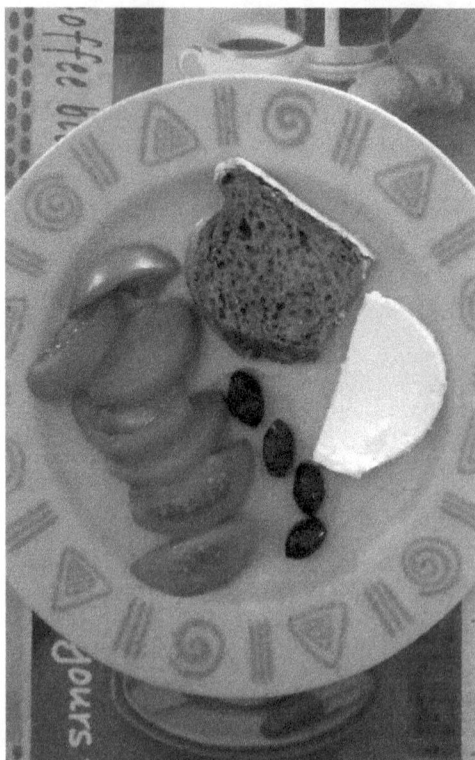

RECIPE 10

SWEET
1 piece of cream cheese

SOUR
Half a tomato

SALTY
1 slice of bread

BITTER
3-4 Olives

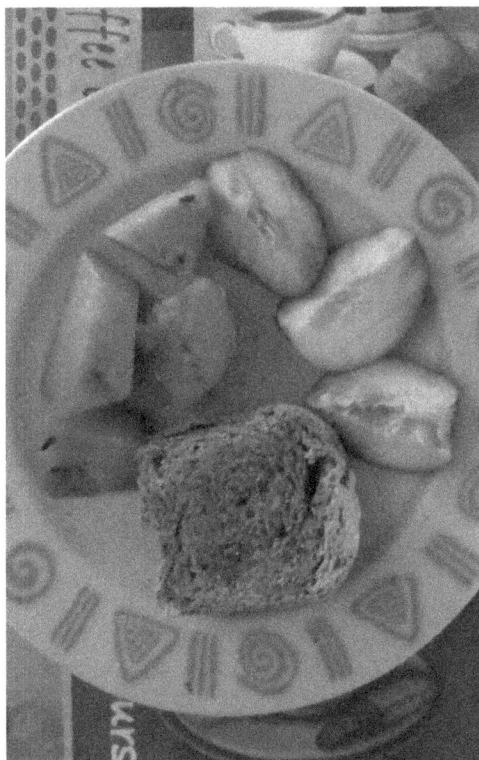

RECIPE 11

SWEET
2 pieces of watermelon

SOUR
1 peach

SALTY
1 slice of bread

BITTER
1 ss of Olive oil with oregano

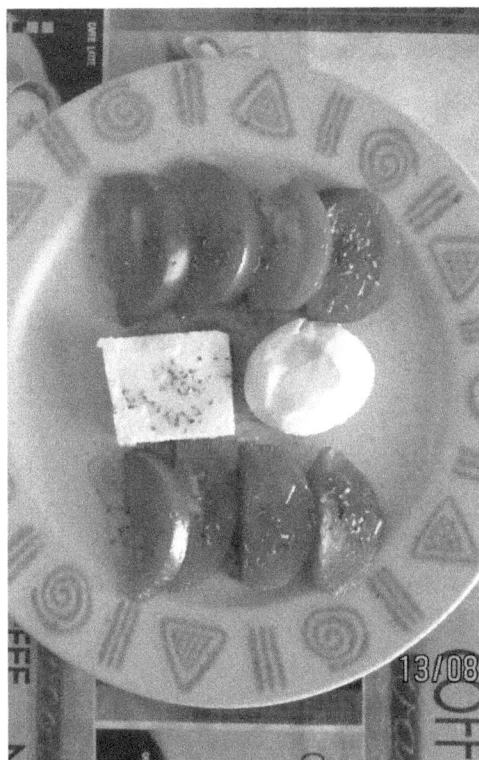

RECIPE 12

SWEET
1 egg

SOUR
Half a tomato

SALTY
1 piece of feta cheese

BITTER
1 ss of olive oil with oregano

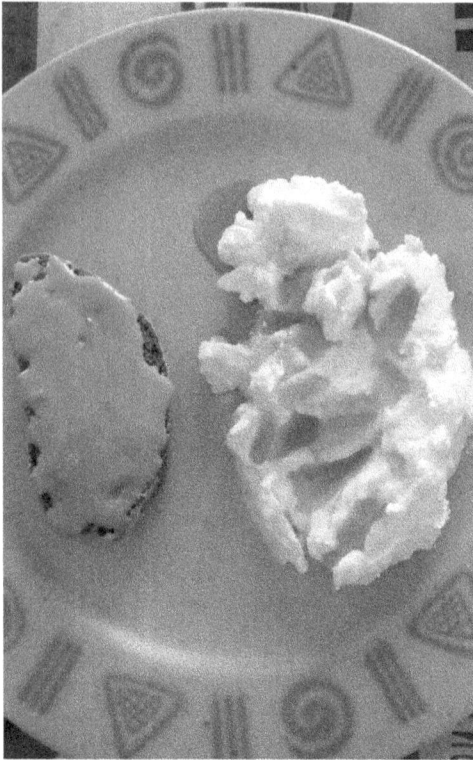

RECIPE 13

SWEET
1 ds of Honey

SOUR
1 Greek yoghurt

SALTY
1 slice of bread

BITTER
1 ss of Tahini

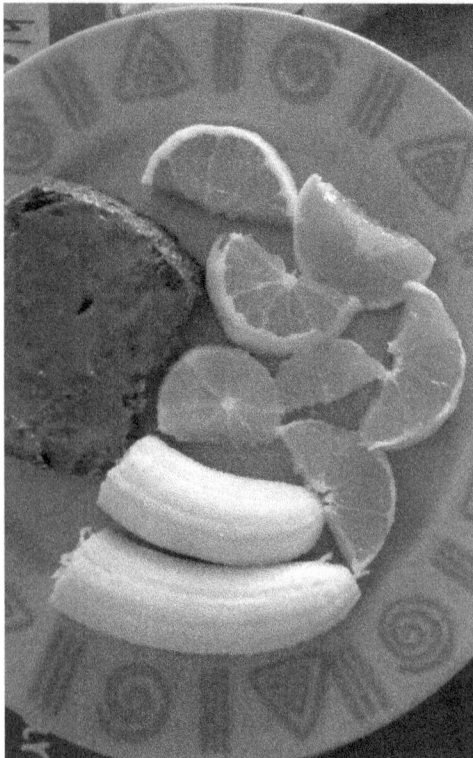

RECIPE 14

SWEET
1 banana

SOUR
1 orange

SALTY
1 slice of bread

BITTER
1 ss of tahini

Note: Bread and rusks can be either salty or sour depending on their methods of preparation.

QUICK GREEK RECIPES FOR LUNCH

(These seven recipes are served on a 20 cm diameter plate for both men and women along with a salad which is served in a salad bowl)

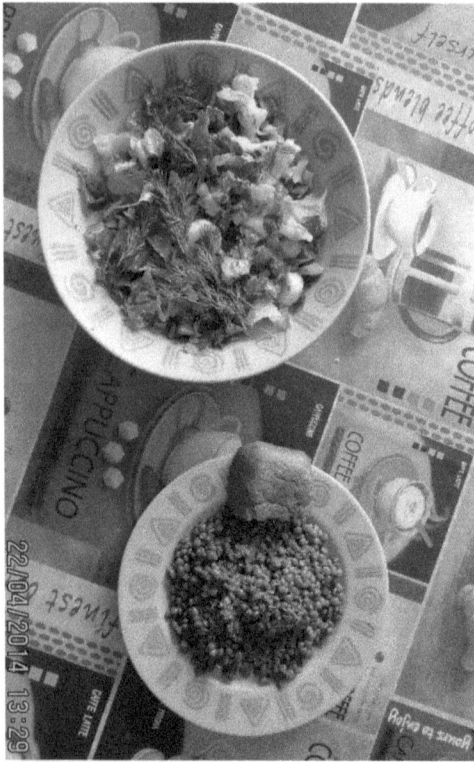

RECIPE 1

ON THE 20 CM PLATE

Sweet – lentils

Salty – bread

IN THE SALAD BOWL

Sour – lemon

Bitter – rocket (arugula), lettuce, oil of oregano

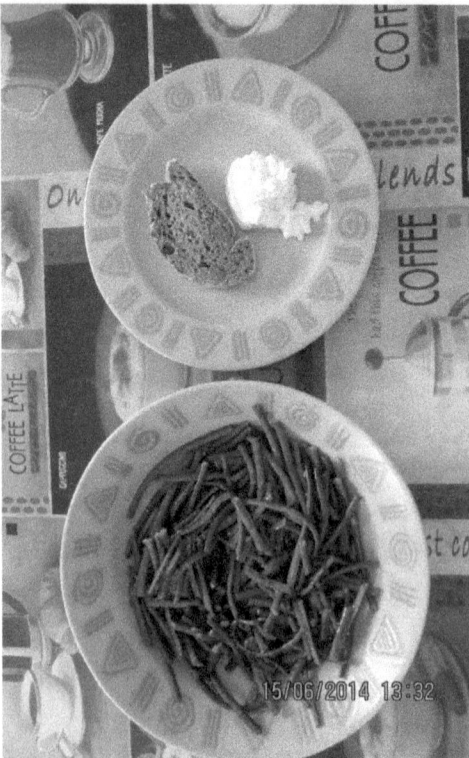

RECIPE 2

ON THE 20 CM PLATE

Salty – cheese

Sour – bread

IN THE SALAD BOWL

Sweet – runner beans

Bitter – oil of oregano

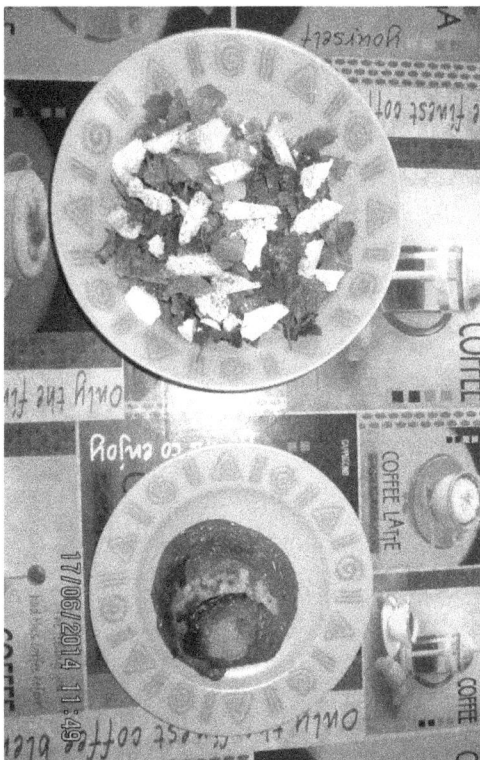

RECIPE 3

ON THE 20 CM PLATE

Sour – tomato
Sweet – rice

IN THE SALAD BOWL

Salty – feta cheese
Bitter – lettuce, arugula, oil of oregano

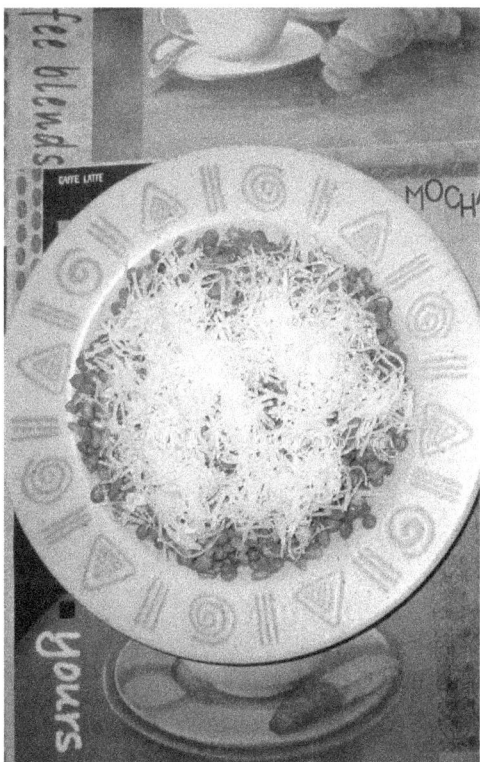

RECIPE 4

ON THE 20 CM PLATE

Sweet – lentils
Salty – cheese

IN THE SALAD BOWL

Sour – lemon
Bitter – lettuce oil of oregano

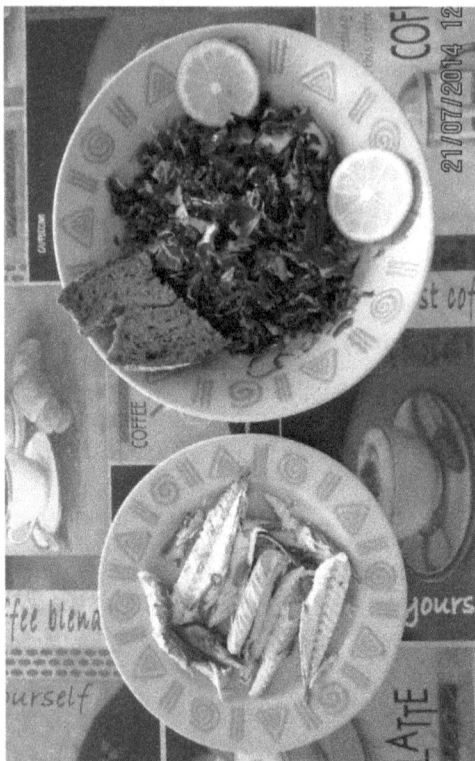

RECIPE 5

ON THE 20 CM PLATE

Sweet – fish

IN THE SALAD BOWL

Bitter – red cabbage
Salty – bread
Sour – lemon

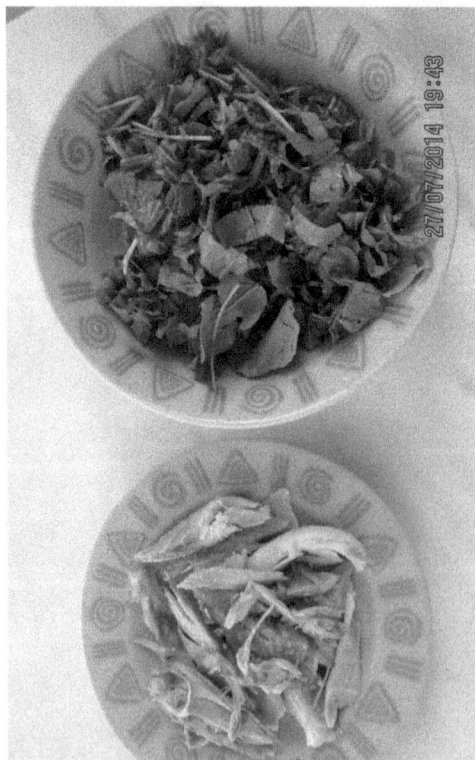

RECIPE 6

ON THE 20 CM PLATE

Sweet – chicken

IN THE SALAD BOWL

Bitter – rocket, oil of oregano
Salty – feta cheese
Sour – bread

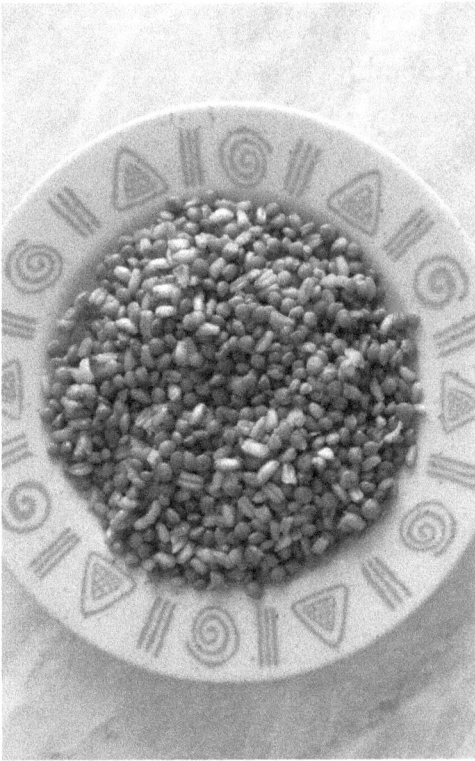

RECIPE 7

ON THE 20 CM PLATE

Sweet – rice, wheat

IN THE SALAD BOWL

Bitter – rocket, oil of oregano
Salty – feta cheese
Sour – bread

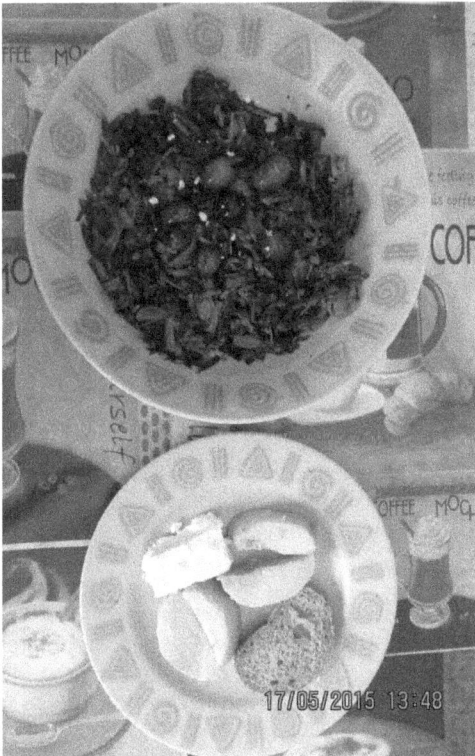

RECIPE 8

ON THE 20 CM PLATE

sweet- potatoes
sour - bread
salty- feta cheese

IN THE SALAD BOWL

Bitter – Wild greens, olives,
olive oil

TABLES OF FOODSTUFFS
(Bitter, Sour, Salty, and Sweet)

And here are the four categories of flavours with some of the foods that belong to these categories.

Bitter tasting foods

Asparagus	Coffee	Mustard (black)	Spinach
Basil	Curly cabbage	Oregano	Swiss chard
Beer	Dill	Parsley	Tahini
Broccoli	Eggplant	Radish	Tea
Brussels sprouts	Endive	Red cabbage	Thyme
Celery	Fennel	Rocket	Watercress
Celery root	Greek beverages	Rosemary	Wild greens
Chocolate drink	Kale	Sage	
Cinnamon	Lettuce	Savory	

Sweet tasting foods

Apple	Leek
Apricot	Lentils
Banana	Lettuce
Beans (broad)	Maize
Beans (common)	Manouri (cheese)
Beans (runner)	Meat
Beetroot	Nectarine
Cantaloupe	Nuts (unsalted)
Carrot	Onion
Cauliflower	Pear
Chickpeas	Pepper
Cucumber	Plums
Dates	Pomegranate
Eggs	Potatoes
Figs	Potatoes (sweet)
Fish	Pumpkin
Fruits (dried)	Raisins
Grapes	Ricotta
Gruyere (cheese)	Swede
Halva	Watermelon
Kasseri (cheese)	

Sour tasting foods

Sour tasting foods	Mizithra (cheese)
Blackberries	Orange
Bread (made from sourdough)	Peach
	Pomegranate
Cherries (sour juice drink)	Rusk (made from sourdough)
Cherries (sour)	Strawberries
Crab apple	Tangerine
Goat's Cheese	Tomato
Grapefruit	Vinegar
Lemon	Yoghurt (Greek)

Salty tasting foods

Bread
Dill
Feta (Greek cheese)
Gruyere (cheese)
Kefalotiri (cheese)
Kopanisti (cheese)
Rusk

A lot of foods can be placed in two categories; this is because there are different varieties of the same food: e.g. some may be sweet and others may be sour. For example, apples can be sweet or sour. The same applies to peaches, pomegranates, and many other fruits: and this phenomenon is equally true for vegetables.

FOR BREAKFAST & DINNER

Sweet tasting foods

Apple
Apricot
Banana
Cantaloupe
Dates
Eggs
Figs
Fruits (dried)
Grapes
Gruyere (cheese)
Honey
Kasseri (cheese)
Manouri (cheese)
Nectarine
Peach
Pear
Plums
Raisins
Ricotta (cheese)
Watermelon

Sour tasting foods

Blackberries
Bread
(made with sourdough)
Cherries
(sour juice drink)
Cherries (sour)
Crab Apple
Goat's cheese
Grapefruit
Lemon
Mizithra (cheese)
Orange
Peach
Pomegranate
Strawberries
Tangerine
Tomato
Yoghurt (Greek)

Salty tasting foods

Bread
Feta (Greek cheese)
Gruyere (cheese)
Kefalotiri (cheese)
Kopanisti (cheese)
Rusk

Bitter tasting foods

Cinnamon
Olive oil
Olives
tahini

FOR LUNCH
(ON THE 20 CM DIAMETER PLATE)

Sweet tasting foods	Salty tasting foods
Beans (broad)	Bread
Beans (common)	Dill
Chickpeas	Feta (Greek cheese)
Eggs	Gruyere (cheese)
Fish	Kefalotiri (cheese)
Gruyere (cheese)	Kopanisti (cheese)
Kasseri (cheese)	Rusk
Lentils	
Manouri (cheese)	
Meat	
Ricotta (cheese)	

FOR THE SALAD BOWL

Bitter tasting foods for the salad	Bitter tasting foods	
Asparagus	Asparagus	Radish
Broccoli	Basil	Red cabbage
Brussels sprouts	Beer	Rocket
Cabbage (curly)	Broccoli	Rosemary
Cabbage (red)	Brussels sprouts	Sage
Celery	Celery	Savory
Celery root	Celery root	Spinach
Eggplant	Chocolate drink	Swiss chard
Endive	Cinnamon	Tahini
Fennel	Coffee	Tea
Greens (wild)	Curly cabbage	Thyme
Kale	Dill	Watercress
Lettuce	Eggplant	
Mustard (black)	Endive	
Parsley	Fennel	
Radish	Greek beverages	
Rocket	Kale	
Spinach	Lettuce	
Swiss chard	Mustard (black)	
Watercress	Oregano	

Sweet tasting foods for the salad	Sour tasting foods for the salad
Beans	Bread (sourdough)
Beetroot	Goat's cheese
Carrot	Lemon
Cauliflower	Mizithra (cheese)
Cucumber	Rusk (made from sourdough)
Leek	Tomato
Lettuce	Vinegar
Maize	
Onion	
Pepper	
Potatoes	
Potatoes (sweet)	
Pumpkin	
Runner beans	
Swede	

For the salad, you can use a variety of bitter flavoured foods.
And to finish off:

Bitter herbs	Bitter Drinks
Basil	Beer
Oregano	Beverages (Greek)
Rosemary	Chocolate drink
Sage	Coffee
Savory	Tea
Thyme	

DINNER

IF YOU ARE REALLY HUNGER, HAVE YOUR BREAKFAST AGAIN: FOR MEN – ON A 25 CM. DIAMETER PLATE AND FOR WOMEN – ON A 20 CM. DIAMETER PLATE. IF YOU ARE REALLY FAMISHED, YOU CAN HAVE YOUR LUNCH AGAIN.

MONDAY

FOOD EATEN – TASTE – REASON FOR EATING IT (HABIT)

Morning

Lunch

Dinner

TUESDAY

FOOD EATEN – TASTE – REASON FOR EATING IT (HABIT)

Morning

Lunch

Dinner

WEDNESDAY

FOOD EATEN – TASTE – REASON FOR EATING IT (HABIT)

Morning

Lunch

Dinner

THURSDAY

FOOD EATEN – TASTE – REASON FOR EATING IT (HABIT)

Morning

Lunch

Dinner

FRIDAY

FOOD EATEN – TASTE – REASON FOR EATING IT (HABIT)

Morning

Lunch

Dinner

SATURDAY

FOOD EATEN – TASTE – REASON FOR EATING IT (HABIT)

Morning

Lunch

Dinner

SUNDAY

Morning

Lunch

Dinner

SEASONING: SALT MIXED WITH HERBS

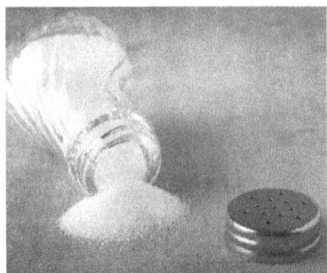

Using a mortar and pestle or a grinding mill, you can prepare your own seasoning of salt mixed with herbs. The herbs must be bought in dry form and the salt must be unrefined, and they should be combined in a ratio of 1:3 – one part salt with three parts herbs. Later, this can be changed to a ratio of 1:5. The mixture should be ground until it has become extremely fine then it can be placed in a cruet and used as a seasoning. After some time – in my case, it was about a month – you may be able to do completely without salt and just use a mixture of ground herbs as a seasoning. Some of the herbs that I use, and which you might like to try, are as follows: nettle, rosemary, lavender, sage, oregano, savory, mint, thyme, spearmint, coriander, cardamom, ginger, pepper, basil, nutmeg, onion, garlic, and bay leaves. Here are five recipes for Greek seasonings which I use with for my meals.

[KEY ds: dessert spoon; ss: soup spoon.]

SEASONING 1
1 ds of salt
1 ss of garlic
1 ss of pepper
1 ss of sage
1 ss of rosemary

SEASONING 2
1 ds of salt
1 ss of celery
1 ss of parsley
1 ss of thyme
1 ss of savory
1 ss of dill
1 ss of basil

SEASONING 3
1 ds of salt
1 ss of thyme
1 ss of savory
1 ss of basil
1 ss of oregano
1 ss of marjoram

SEASONING 4
1 ds of salt
1 ss of mint
1 ss of oregano
1 ss of rosemary
1 ss of marjoram
1 ss of tomato

SEASONING 5
1 ds of salt
1 ss of oregano
1 ss of daphne
1 ss of rosemary
1 ss of tomato

Thanks to

Still in 2015 there still are true friends! I wish to extend my warmest thanks to Michalis Antonopoulos, Othon Gkotsis and Notis Rigas, who worked with artistry and love for the book cover, paging and charts.
Sokratis, Loukia, Dionysia, Panayiotis, George, Nick, Marie-Paul, and Polyxeni provided valuable insight to the content of the book.

www.ingramcontent.com/pod-product-compliance
Lightning Source LLC
Chambersburg PA
CBHW062145020426
42334CB00020B/2518